11/8/04

To Barbara
Bet wissen ...
continued successful life!

Alan M

life's a
smelling
SUCCESS

using scent to empower
your memory and learning

DR. ALAN HIRSCH, M.D.

Authors of Unity Publishing ✦ New York

Authors of Unity Publishing
575 Madison Ave.
10th Floor
New York, NY 10022
(212) 605-0407
www.authorsofunity.com

Book design by Sara Patton
Back cover copy by Susan Kendrick Writing
Printed in the USA
Second printing

PUBLISHER'S CATALOGING-IN-PUBLICATION
(Provided by Quality Books, Inc.)

Hirsch, Alan R.
  Life's a smelling success : using scent to empower
your memory and learning / Alan Hirsch.
    p. cm.
    LCCN 2002114983
    ISBN 0-9725250-1-7

  1. Smell. 2. Memory—Physiological aspects.
3. Odors. 4. Aromatherapy. I. Title.

QP458.H57 2003   153.1'2
                        QBI33-874

Contents

Acknowledgments

There are many I wish to thank for their help and assistance in completing this book.

Thanks to Dr. Jan Fawcett and Dr. Jacob Fox of the Rush-Presbyterian-St. Luke's Medical Center, Chicago, for their teaching and encouragement over the years.

I wish to acknowledge Stanley Block for his many hours of guidance.

This project could not have been completed without the efforts of Denise Fahey, Genie Gurgone, and Virginia McCollough.

To my wife, Debra. Without her understanding and many sacrifices, I would never have been able to undertake this project.

Thank you all!

To my family, loving and understanding,
whose joy and playfulness today create
tomorrow's happiest memories.

Foreword

I met Alan Hirsch while walking in the Italian countryside. Dr. Hirsch is a neurologist, psychiatrist, marathon runner, and the author of *Dr. Hirsch's Guide to Scentsational Weight Loss, Scentsational Sex,* and *What Flavor Is Your Personality?*

Our Italian adventure with the Hirsches led to other trips, including one to Egypt, where we saw Cairo, the Sphinx, and climbed a narrow tunnel full of ghosts inside one of the pyramids—then up the Nile on a Sheraton boat to see many other remains of the Pharaoh's ancient civilization.

Egypt is interesting, and we had a good time ... until disaster struck. We had been warned to drink only bottled water, and Alan, a doctor, brought pills for protection—but those precautions weren't enough. He had given away his supply to the other tourists. He got painfully ill, and then my wife did too. The Egyptians were kind and did what they could, but I took her out of the country in a wheelchair. At the airport, a giant mobile elevator made by Mercedes-Benz lifted her to the door of the plane, wheelchair and all.

I have a keen memory for the past. I remember Egypt as if it were just yesterday, not a decade ago. It's my memory for the present that isn't so great ... my memory apparatus leaves much to be desired. I know a bad memory can be fixed. I know because I experienced an improvement—temporarily, for a year or two, long, long ago. Most improvement techniques were complicated and began to take over my life.

That's why Dr. Hirsch's book is so wonderful. This is not tough stuff. Actually, it is more like fun. What we have here are easy ways to sharpen your memory—remember your wedding anniversary, your neighbor's names, your mom's birthday, and what you were supposed to bring home for dinner. You'll even remember where you left your keys and eyeglasses. This book enabled me to start adopting some of Dr. Hirsch's suggestions (he has many) to improve my memory.

There are more good ideas in this book than you can use. The writing is light and joyful—astonishing for a scientist. He is truly a masterful writer.

This is a pleasurable book that can change your whole life for the better. Enjoy!

– Henry C. Cowen, CEO,
The Cowen Group, and author of
I Sent You A Letter . . . Did You Reply?
(True Tales of a Junk Mail Whiz)
Trafford Publishing, Victoria, BC, Canada, 2001

A Note to the Reader

Although scientists have not yet unlocked the ultimate mystery of memory, we do know that remembering and forgetting are the province of the brain. The more we understand about the way the brain works, the more we can improve our ability to learn and retain information. I wrote *Life's a Smelling Success* to share with you the fundamental principles of memory and learning and then link this information with the latest research about ways in which your sense of smell can help you learn faster and retain more.

Memory devices are not new. For centuries, philosophers, psychologists, educators, and scientists have attempted to explain memory and have created formulas to improve memory. However, this is the first book that explores the way the sense of smell can influence our ability to absorb and recall what we want and need to know. In addition, offered free with this book is an odorized bookmark, using the floral scent The Smell & Taste Treatment and Research Foundation has used in learning research and is available in Baby Boom's SmartScents toy line to enhance infant brain development. After reading the first chapter of this book, you can begin to use the bookmark immediately for your own learning and performance applications.

Every known culture has used odors as an integral part of their traditions and rituals. Poets and other writers have described the sense of smell as the "memory" sense, perhaps because of the universal link between odors and nostalgia. Nothing brings back memories of the past as quickly as an odor, a phenomenon known as *olfactory-evoked recall*. This phenomenon influences the way we respond to a variety of experiences and may play a role in helping us understand the relationship between mood and memory. Nostalgia has particular relevance here because once we understand it, we can concentrate on evaluating the kinds of memories we, through our actions, are creating today.

In addition, *Life's a Smelling Success* explores the reasons we forget as well as the variety of ways we remember. I also explore the concept of malodor—unpleasant smells and their negative effect on memory and learning. In addition, I discuss "social memory," which involves the way you remember others and the way others remember you. We all give and receive "scent impressions" every day, and these impressions become woven with other information we have about individuals we encounter. You will also find a new memory device, the "Odorbet," which will help you remember names of new people you meet.

For more than 100 years, popular aromatherapists have attempted to improve health and alter mood with scents, and this book presents research about the potential for medical application of various odors. The continuing ability to learn and retain information is of particular interest among the "baby boom" population, as well as their elderly parents. For this reason, I included advice about keeping brainpower and memory sharp over a lifetime. For example, a strong link exists between physical health and mental abilities; based on current research, engaging in regular exercise is the best, and probably least expensive, insurance policy for preserving memory and the ability to learn and analyze new information.

Life's a Smelling Success also addresses concerns of parents and their children. In addition to exploring research that links odors and learning, I also discuss issues that influence learning, including ways to affect attention span and the kind of sensory-rich environment in which children thrive.

You will also find a variety of exercises and memory tips throughout the book. Some use odors and some do not, but all are designed for men and women of all ages who wish to make the most of their mental abilities and gifts and to strengthen and preserve them over a lifetime.

– Alan R. Hirsch, M.D.
Smell & Taste Treatment and Research Foundation
Chicago, Illinois • October 2002

The Mysterious Goddess of Memory

The wisest man I ever knew taught me something I never forgot. And although I never forgot it, I never quite memorized it either. So what I'm left with is the memory of having learned something very wise that I can't quite remember.

— George Carlin, *Braindroppings*

In the last few years, our sense of smell has gained enormous new respect, and we have entered what we can legitimately call the "Golden Age" of the nose. Perhaps the recent attention given to the power of odors has provided you with a new understanding of the ways of the once-forgotten sense of smell. The attention is well placed because recent research confirms that your nose is far more important to your well being and enjoyment of life than once believed.

Today, a variety of odors have myriad uses. We can use scents to lift our mood or help us sleep; certain smells appear to help curb appetite, making the nose a partner in attempts to achieve a healthful weight. And we cannot forget the well-publicized research that links specific odors with sexual arousal in both men and women. We also are making progress in developing safe, non-invasive "odor therapies" to enhance health and, perhaps one day, aromatherapy based on scientific research will become a routine component of treatment for health concerns such as migraine headaches and mild anxiety disorders.

Scents and fragrances are of great economic importance, and monetary considerations form a powerful engine to drive commercial research. The aromas you inhale in the shopping mall or café do not appear accidentally. Millions of dollars are spent on market testing before a new perfume or cologne is released, and even the most basic products such as deodorant and mouthwash are carefully designed to include odors that appeal to large numbers of people. Research confirms that odors even influence the traffic pattern in casinos and how long individuals play at a particular slot machine!

Perhaps one of the important, and most practical, areas of current interest involves the role of odors in memory and learning. These areas of universal interest take on importance because the growing population of older adults is eager to find ways to preserve memory and stay mentally fit. In addition, parents currently show great interest in enhancing educational environments for young people.

Based on what we already know about the relationship of the sense of smell with memory and learning, I predict that by the year 2010 or so it will be a common practice to add specific odors to the classroom environment. Eventually, teachers will use different types of smells to enhance different kinds of learning, so the odors introduced during math class may be different from odors used for art and music instruction. The practice will extend to factories and offices, and we won't ignore our homes when we add scents to improve our memory and help us learn and retain new information. You can use this book and begin adding "productive" odors to your own environment. But the odors you use in your living room to induce relaxation may be different from the scents you add to your home office while you work on your tax returns or prepare for a test.

We Are Always Learning

Many methods exist to enhance memory with odors and also help you learn new information. What exactly is a learning environment? A learning environment can be defined as a classroom, of course, or an office, but even a cocktail party or a professional networking meeting can serve as a setting where you need and want to learn. When you struggle to remember the names of people you meet, you are immersed in a learning environment, just as taking a line dancing class and studying a how-to book on childcare or plumbing represent learning environments, too. Hearing a phone number for the first time is a learning experience if you want to remember it. If you don't, it's just another bit of trivia that you allow to "go in one ear and out the other."

We can view memory in a purely practical way and discuss it in terms of facts and skills and the lasting impressions of people, places, and things we carry around in our brains. But the more poetic among us may prefer memory's mysterious and ethereal qualities. Consider that the word *memory* itself comes from Greek mythology. Mnemosyne is the goddess who, as a result of adulterous encounters with Zeus, gave birth to the nine Muses, the nine qualities of imagination. Mnemosyne rules the world of memory and education, and her legacy is found in the language of remembering. A mnemonic device is a system or even a trick devised to help us remember something important. And according to the myth, when we forget something, we have fallen into the river Lethe, the waters of forgetfulness.

Mnemosyne Lives in the Brain

Poetry aside, memory is the province of the brain. We all have a personal Mnemosyne — and her children the Muses — that reside in different regions of the brain. It is the brain that stores our personal joys and sorrows as well as the mundane scripts we use every day to drive a car or turn on a light in the kitchen. When the brain's complex mechanisms work well, we add new information and retrieve data stored over a lifetime or for a minute or two. Ultimately, the brain controls what we remember and what we forget, and throughout this book I discuss brain mechanisms that regulate how we retain and recall information from sensory cues. However, we don't need to understand the brain's intricate systems before we begin using them to enhance our ability to retain and recall information that is important to us.

The Nose Remembers, Too

Since the early days of human development, our sense of smell helps us avoid danger and find fresh food and protects us from consuming spoiled food. Just as the sensation of pain protects the body from injury and provides a signal that something is wrong, our sense of smell protects us from harm, too. Imagine how dangerous life would be if we had no odor memory. What if each time we detected a gas odor we had to learn it was potentially lethal? What if we couldn't identify the odor of smoke? Association between odors and memory represent one of our most important protective mechanisms and even in our high-tech culture remains critical for the survival of our species. We also are beginning to understand that odors can directly help us learn new information, and one way we can do this is by using the principles of a concept called state-dependent learning.

Names and Dates and Chocolate

We often overlook the importance of *state-dependent learning*, which is one of the most basic learning and memory concepts.

The mechanism is actually quite simple. In order to improve our ability to retrieve information, we should duplicate the state, or condition, that was present at the time we learned the information. For example, if you eat chocolate while studying for a history test, the chocolate becomes a *contextual cue.* Your ability to recall the information will be enhanced if you eat chocolate when you enter the classroom.

Both internal and external cues play a role in linking a substance such as chocolate to learning. The *external* cue is the chocolate itself, and it becomes a feature of the environment. The *internal* cues involve the sugar rush and the taste and smell of the chocolate. So, when you nibble on a chocolate candy bar before taking your test, you are duplicating the internal and external cues.

Of course, chocolate represents just one example, and I'm not necessarily recommending that you eat candy when you are attempting to learn. The odor and taste of coffee or tea—or carrots—may also serve as both an internal and external contextual cue. Contextual cues can include many things, including location. Ideally, you should study for a test or work on particular project in the same environment again and again. Writers, for example, are often told to choose a special place to write every day, and that place becomes associated with creativity and productivity. It is as if the brain is trained to respond again and again to the same external cues. Students are often told to study in the same place every day in order to improve their concentration and recall.

As unusual as it sounds, an underwater environment can even serve as a contextual cue. In the 1970s, an experiment was conducted that involved learning a list of words, either while on the beach or fifteen feet below the surface of the water. Participants learned lists of words equally well in both environments.

However, the contextual cues were important. The words learned under water were better recalled under water; the words learned on the beach were better recalled on the beach. In fact, the participants recalled 40 percent fewer words when the learning and recall environments were switched.

Contextual cues may also include mental and physical states. Most medical interns are tired much of the time because they are expected to be on duty for many hours, and their sleep (when they can find time to rest) is often interrupted. However, these interns learn significant amounts of information when they are tired, and hence may recall it more readily when they are tired, a state that functions as an internal cue. Likewise, studies have shown that if you learn something when you're drunk, it is easier to recall it after you have been drinking. The inebriated state is an internal cue. Since both extreme fatigue and excessive consumption of alcohol are detrimental to health, not to mention intellectual functioning, over the long term *don't* fix yourself a drink when you want to learn history or math. But this information provides a clear example of state-dependent learning and healthier ways exist to enhance learning. You can begin using state-dependent learning techniques immediately; no long learning curve is necessary.

You *Can* Remember Names

If you are trying to recall a name, start by trying to remember other internal or external cues. Let's say that you met a person at a cocktail party when you were tired and hungry. You know you were wearing your favorite cologne because you always wear that fragrance on social occasions. Then you try to recall the person's face and clothing or other features, including his or her cologne. If you were standing when you met this person, then stand up and walk around when you are trying to recall the name. Recalling the surroundings helps to remember other details about an event. This is an example of using a kinesthetic memory to enhance recall. Likewise, try to remember your mood state. Were you happy or bored? All these cues may help you retrieve the name—if you learned it in the first place. This is an important point: *You can't recall what you don't know.*

When you use these techniques to recall information, you are using the same principles interns and underwater divers used to remember information. This is classic state-dependent learning, and we can add another element to encourage even greater retention and recall.

Can Peppermint and Butterscotch Make Us Smarter?

In 1995, the Smell & Taste Treatment and Research Foundation formed a coalition with *Super Science,* a magazine published by Scholastic Magazine. Sixth-grade students were given word lists to memorize in the presence of the odor of either butterscotch or peppermint candy and also when no odor was introduced into the environment.

We found that students retained more words when the same odor used during learning was introduced during retrieval, the time at which children were asked to remember the words. When a different odor was introduced, the children were unable to recall the same number of words. The peppermint or butterscotch odors served as contextual cues and enhanced the ability of the children to recall the memorized words.

In this study, butterscotch produced better "word scholars" than peppermint, which raises the question about special attributes or characteristics of specific odors. In this case, however, I do not believe we have a great mystery on our hands. While butterscotch is a common odor, children are exposed to peppermint more often and hence it had less effect. If children brushed their teeth with butterscotch-flavored toothpaste, then that odor may have been less effective too. As with all sensory stimuli, the novelty effect operates with odors. The effectiveness of any external odor eventually diminishes, and the odor of butterscotch could have eventually become less effective if we introduced it many times. Peppermint is not a novel odor for most children, so even though it induces an alert mental state, it did not have the same "power" as the less familiar odor of butterscotch.

It is important to recognize, however, that introducing a specific odor to a classroom task enhanced performance. Our study suggests that perhaps our schools are missing an important link to memory and learning if they ignore the impact of odors on state-dependent learning. Equally important, we don't need to be sixth graders to benefit from this information. We can all use odors to improve our brainpower.

The bookmark you ordered with this book is designed to help you use a tested odor to help you learn, retain, and recall information. You can use this odor to create a state-dependent learning environment, much like we created with a group of adult volunteers.

Sniffing the Floral Odors

In 1995, our foundation conducted a study that measured the ability of 22 research participants (12 men, 10 women) to complete the trail-making subtest of the Halsted-Reitan Test Battery, which is a standard psychological test that measures a wide range of mental abilities. (The trail-making subtest involves connecting a series of numbers.) Screening tests had established that these individuals had a normal ability to smell and normal learning ability. We gave the test in both the presence and the absence of a mixed floral odor.

On average, subjects were able to complete the test *17 percent faster* in the presence of the odor. We had originally hypothesized that the presence of any odor that was considered pleasant would improve performance. However, our early pilot tests did not support this hypothesis. For example, odors such as baked goods, lavender, citrus, parsley, and spearmint did not improve learning speed, even though in the pilot studies individuals considered these odors positive. We used some of these odors in other contexts and they have shown specific effects on mood or behavior. For example, lavender enhances alpha waves in the back of the head and induces relaxation and may promote sleep. When combined with pumpkin pie, lavender was the top-performing odor in our male sexual arousal study. The odor of baked goods triggers the olfactory-evoked nostalgia response in a large percentage of adults. In other words, a whiff of freshly baked bread or pastries may instantly take us on a memory journey to the past. Based on our testing, neither the odor of baked goods or lavender has the ability to enhance learning, but the floral odor embedded in your bookmark can.

Later in this book, I offer a more detailed discussion about the ways we think the floral odor may enhance learning, even though we can't yet pinpoint the neurophysiologic mechanism that would provide a specific explanation. In a sense, almost all the information presented here will help you understand why and how odors act on the brain and influence mood, behavior, learning, and performance.

I Feel Good, Therefore I Perform Well

Although odors may have a specific effect on the brain, we know that fragrances that lift moods may positively influence learning, memory, and performance. It's certainly possible that the individuals in our study experienced a subtle mood change in the presence of the odor because they liked it. Had we introduced an unpleasant smell, it is probable that the performance of the men and women would have decreased. The same principle operated when we introduced butterscotch and peppermint odors to the children in a classroom setting. The students liked the odor and they probably felt a "lift" when the odor was introduced.

Anatomically, the olfactory system is part of the limbic brain, the center of emotional life. Positive and negative responses to odors are immediate and occur before the odor is identified. The men and women in our study may have had a positive reaction to the odor, which affected their mood and perhaps even caused a nostalgic response, which generally enhances one's mood in a positive way.

We also know that anxiety inhibits learning. There is a delicate balance between relaxation and alert attention. The odor of lavender, which has been shown to induce a relaxed mood, actually impaired performance on arithmetic tasks, a *left-brain* activity, perhaps because study participants became too relaxed. But we can speculate that lavender may be appropriate for *right-brain* activities such as listening to music or painting. We already know that the odor of lavender has a positive effect on male sexual arousal, and sex is certainly a right-brain activity.

A Task of Your Own

Start experimenting with the power of scents to help learn or work more quickly and with greater focus by using the scented bookmark offered free with this book. Pick a task, any task that you repeat and in which you need accuracy and concentration. Sniff the bookmark and keep it near you while you balance your checkbook, study for a test, or work on a specific type of project for your job, one that you repeat on a regular basis. You may try using the odor in a setting where you are learning a new skill, such as mastering a new computer program or studying a foreign language.

Each time you work on this task, you can use the odor, thereby creating a state-dependent learning environment. Each time you sniff the fragrance and work on your task, you reinforce its usefulness. You may notice a difference if you forget to sniff! Over time, you will begin to associate the mixed floral odor with the particular task, and you may miss it if you forget. Choose a different odor to use with a different type of task. Throughout this book, I will talk about the kinds of smells that influence different moods and behavior, and this information will help you build your own "odor library."

We Learn What We Need to Know

Every day — usually without laborious effort — we perform hundreds of tasks and sort through volumes of data stored in our brain. Many of our actions resemble what Roger Schank, a theorist in the field of artificial intelligence, calls "scripts." These scripts combine experiences and expectations and produce automatic responses. If you take the train to work each morning, you understand and remember the sequence of steps it takes to get you to the station and what is necessary to find a seat and settle in. You are responding in habitual ways to familiar sensory information and procedures. This is an automatic process, interrupted only by an event that makes everything different. For example, boarding the right train in Tokyo or Moscow may require conscious thought processes. Your mental concepts of ticket, platform, train car, and seat will now adapt to an unfamiliar set of circumstances. And it is likely that you will not soon forget your first subway ride in a foreign country.

We think about our memory when we forget, usually

momentarily, who was the president 12 years ago or what happened in a mystery novel we loved so much. (How could we forget those plot twists and characters?) We know we have a storehouse of memories, but we often don't understand why we remember scores of seemingly useless facts and, equally important, why we forget, even for a second or two, information or events that seem critical at that moment.

The Central Questions

It is easy to see why the world of Mnemosyne is mysterious and intriguing, even though modern science has made progress in identifying regions in the brain that control different types of memory and physical and mental functions. The basic questions that have puzzled humans for centuries remain: Why do we remember, and equally important, why do we forget? Why do we remember the trivial and forget the important? Most of us believe that we *should* remember the Latin verb forms we studied in high school and the name of Argentina's president. Didn't we just read about him in the newspaper the other day?

We must also ask how we are able to forget. We are deluged with volumes of information every day, and if we were to remember it all we would be overwhelmed—we would literally overload our 100 billion brain cells. Even before the so-called Information Revolution, it was imperative that we possess the ability to ignore stimuli and select what will "imprint" on the memory centers of the brain. In fact, many of us spend time becoming frustrated over the inability to remember things that we never knew in the first place! On other occasions, we remember things we forgot we ever knew.

One theory of memory is that everything we see, hear, smell, taste, and touch records as a memory and transfers to storage in the brain. So, even if we do not consciously remember the color of the carpet in our first apartment, that information is stored in the brain, along with other less than earth-shattering data, like every crack on the sidewalk of every street we've walked upon. Sigmund Freud, who believed lapses of memory were indicative of repressed memory, adopted this theory. His statement that "in mental life nothing which has once been formed can perish" illustrates this theory.

Another theory is that only selected material is encoded in the brain. What we pay attention to stays with us and what has emotional impact is recorded. In addition, the brain is influenced by what kind of learning is encouraged and used, and the topography of the brain reflects ongoing changes in information stored and used. In addition, much of what we remember may be *integrated memories*, a collage of disparate memories all clumped together, rather than accurate recollections of individual experiences. Behavioral studies tend to support the theory that memory is selective and fluid rather than static. Either way, we are always in the process of evaluating what we want and need to remember and what we neither need nor want to retain.

Our Sense of Smell Is Our Memory's Friend

In this book, you will learn about memory in general, but also about the anatomic and neurochemical overlap between the sense of smell and memory. You probably are already aware of the close link between odors and emotions. If a whiff of a particular odor is sufficient to send you on a nostalgic trip deep into your past, then is it logical to introduce odors into a variety of learning environments? Do odors have the power to help us retain and recall information? I will discuss this in detail because recent information gives us a scientific basis for attempting to enhance learning and memory with odors and through odor association.

The most basic way to view memory is as *an intricate system to store and retrieve previously learned information and experience.* The experience could be as remote as a childhood birthday party or as recent as the weather report you heard during a news show ten minutes ago. The ability to dunk a basketball or perform the *pas de deux* from *Swan Lake* represents another type of memory that can be retrieved on demand. The emotions about an event are remembered too. In fact, the memories surrounding a childhood birthday party are probably so vivid because of the emotional memories, pleasant or unpleasant, embedded in the experience.

Identity and Memory

Humans are different from other animal species, not only because of the volumes of information we can store and our ability to reason, but also because of our unique ability to think about what we know. Our thought processes quite literally change our memories. In addition, our ability to evaluate experience invariably alters our memories and makes us conscious of ourselves. It is often said that our consciousness of self is what differentiates us from other species, even the higher primates. This consciousness of self is in large part dependent on memory. The French philosopher Rene Descartes said, "I think, therefore, I am," but perhaps the more accurate way to express this is, "I remember and I think about what I remember, therefore I am." The "I" of each of us is dependent on our memories. This consciousness of self also allows us to think about the past and make plans for the future.

The sense of "we" is dependent on memory, too. What are holidays if not a way in which we acknowledge collective memory? The shared experience of holidays strengthens the sense of belonging and connection to others. Both our sense of individuality and the sense of being part of a culture are possible because of shared—or collective—memories.

The field of psychiatry is largely the study of the human ability to learn and act on or think about what is known. In a way, it is the study of memory and how memory affects individual behavior. We know, for example, that memory is about more than just brain cells. What we remember and what we forget is influenced by our mood, emotions, and physical condition as well as by the environment or context (including the odor environment), our evaluation of the importance of a fact or an event, and past experiences and memories.

The Myriad Forms of Learning and Memory

Our experiences have limited meaning if we are unable to remember them. As you will see, there are many different types of memories and classifications for memories. Much of this book is focused on the way memory works and on how you can improve your capacity to learn and remember. My medical and scientific specialties are neurology and psychiatry, with a specific interest in olfaction (the sense of smell), so I include information from studies we have conducted at The Smell & Taste Treatment and Research Foundation in Chicago, along with data gathered from other researchers. It is unfortunate, but true, that much of what scientists know about memory and the brain has been discovered by studying patients who have, in one way or another, experienced loss of memory functioning through illness or trauma to the brain. On the positive side, much of what we know about improving or restoring memory and learning ability comes from the experiences of patients who have recovered these functions after illness or trauma.

If you are interested in improving your learning ability and your memory, there are a few general principles to note and remember. Keep them in mind as you read this book and discover ways to use your nose—and other senses—to keep your memory sharp. The principles listed below certainly seem reasonable and logical, but they also have been scientifically proven to be valid.

1. *Fatigue is detrimental to learning and memory.* When we urge children to get adequate rest before a test, we may sound like nagging parents, but we're imparting great wisdom. The same advice applies to adults.

2. *Motivation to learn and remember is essential to learning and memory.* We remember our first love and forget algebra because we are motivated to remember the pleasant experiences of being in love for the first time, and we may even recall the odors surrounding the experience. For most people, dry facts not associated with emotions and a sensory-rich environment do not provide sufficient motivation for memory retention.

3. *Memories change over time.* For the most part, our memories become more pleasant as time goes on. We have a natural tendency to see the past through "rose-colored glasses." We also add or subtract details to memories, and our attitudes and feelings about an experience change over time. In *A Child's Christmas in Wales*, poet Dylan Thomas describes childhood Christmases that were much the same year after year. He tells readers that his memories have blended together so well that he can't remember if it snowed six days and six nights when he was twelve or if it snowed twelve days and twelve nights when he was six.

4. *Suppressing memories takes great mental energy.* Attempting to forget unpleasant experiences can lead to difficulty with concentration and retention of other experiences. Psychotherapy can help individuals redirect mental energy once expended in attempts to forget certain memories to more life-enriching activities.

5. *Distraction is the memory's enemy.* Many people say that their memory is like a sieve. This is usually an exaggeration, of course, but it is also unrealistic to attempt to remember a name or a phone number when the television is blaring, the phone is ringing, and your three-year-old locked himself in the bathroom. If you can recall the numbers "911," consider yourself accomplished.

6. *You can't recall what you never knew in the first place.* Have you ever searched your brain for the name of a person you are sure you met at a party? Now she's walking toward you in the grocery store and you are drawing a complete blank on her name. Instead of fretting that you're getting older and your memory is shot or that you're too young to be so forgetful, consider the possibility that you never learned that person's name. Sure, you may have heard it, but it slipped away before you ever "recorded" it. Oliver Wendell Holmes said it best: "A man must get a thing before he can forget it."

7. *Learning ability and memory must be used in order to grow in capacity.* Memory is analogous to muscle strength. If we do not exercise a muscle it will atrophy, and *our minds must be exercised to stay sharp, too.* While there is some decline of memory "sharpness" as we age, the more we challenge our mind, the sharper it is likely to stay. When it comes to memory, "use it or lose it" is a good adage to remember.

8. *Physical exercise improves memory.* Studies have shown that individuals who exercise regularly have better memory and capacity for learning than those who do not engage in regular physical activities. Exercise brings more oxygen to the brain, and a well-oxygenated brain is a more efficient brain. This is important for everyone, but may have special significance to the elderly, some of whom may be tempted to stop exercising. Many other benefits to exercise are important, too, but the link

between memory and activity may stick as the incentive you need to start or continue a regular exercise program. Your memory may depend on it.

9. *Odors have the power to trigger memories—especially emotionally important memories—more than any other sense.* As Rudyard Kipling said, "Smells are surer than sights and sounds to make your heart-strings crack." This is good news when the memories are sweet, even bittersweet, or generally pleasant. When odors have the power to dredge up things from the past that we would just as soon not remember, then the experience can be distressing. However, this phenomenon is not something we have control over, and once we understand it, we can use odors to help us remember information that is valuable to us.

10. *Odors can enhance or detract from learning and working environments.* You already know that odors can improve learning, even though we do not know the exact mechanism. On the other hand, *malodors* (bad odors) can actually detract from a learning environment because they distract us, but also because bad odors have the potential to increase aggression, something we definitely do not want in classrooms, offices, and factories. Because odors influence mood, and emotional state influences memory and learning, it appears that the sense of smell has not yet been given its due in any environment in which memory plays a role—and that covers considerable ground.

Memory Is a Popular Topic Today

Books about improving memory are more in demand than ever. With increased knowledge about the aging process and the medical successes in extending the average lifespan, current interest in memory is intensifying. However, we could say that current interest in memory is in actuality a concern about forgetfulness. In June of 1998, *Newsweek* magazine featured memory as a cover story, claiming that "forgetfulness is America's latest health obsession" fostered by the aging baby boomers, who have added mental fitness to physical fitness in their list of life goals.

Consider books such as *Cultural Literacy* by E.D. Hirsch Jr., which includes a daunting list of over 4,500 items of information that, at least according to the author, we must know if we want to consider ourselves socially literate. And the books written for adults that tell us the 1001 things we need to know about this or that subject would give anyone intellectual jitters. The Information Age can seem like the Demanding Age; most of us want to be informed, but we cannot possibly keep up with new information in every field, even those that interest us the most. Then, too, information is not the same as knowledge and knowledge is most certainly not synonymous with wisdom. Information is data, but what we do with the data we collect determines our quality of life.

Another reason for the current interest in memory arises from the rapid expansion of knowledge about the brain itself. The '90s were even called "The Decade of the Brain." Since the key to memory begins with understanding the brain, the next chapter describes some fundamental information about the brain and the olfactory connection to memory. Meanwhile, keep using your bookmark! (See the Products section at the end of the book to learn how to obtain more of the odor.)

2

The Landscape of the Brain

If I had to make a bet I would say that the mind is a ghost from God that comes from the sky and lives in the brain.

— Jimmy Breslin

To understand memory, we need to take a trip through the brain and discuss its various components, which reflect the evolutionary journey of human development. The simplest functions, such as sleeping and eating, to the most complex, such as deciphering mathematical codes or pondering the thoughts of ancient philosophers, are the domain of different regions of the brain. Although we can gain some understanding of the brain by examining its "pieces," we should never stray from the reality that the brain is a well-integrated group of mechanisms, with many functions occurring simultaneously. This is the reason we can eat, talk, watch the news, and think about the movie we're planning to rent later all at the same time. (This may not be advisable, but the brain allows us to carry out this kind of frenzied activity.)

Different regions of the brain are involved in different types of memory and the classifications of memory that I will discuss later. To fully understand both normal and impaired memory, as well as ways to improve memory, you need a rudimentary grasp of the complex workings of the brain. If you can visualize the parts of the brain involved in the thousands of functions you take for granted, the classifications of memory and problems with storage and retrieval will make more sense.

The So-Called Lower Functions

The oldest and most primitive component of brain is its *stem*, which protrudes from the top of the spinal column (see figure 1). In evolutionary terms, the brainstem is what is left of the reptilian brain, but that doesn't mean that it is not critical to survival. The brainstem is involved with essential processes such as breathing and regulating the heartbeat and blood pressure. We don't think about the brainstem, but we can't survive without it.

The *cerebellum*, which literally means "little brain," is located behind the brainstem (see figure 2). The cerebellum is involved with movement and balance. Our muscles and joints depend on the cerebellum to control and monitor their movement. Our learned motor abilities—walking, skiing, swinging a golf club, skipping rope, and riding a bicycle—are stored in the cerebellum.

The *limbic* portion of the brain is located on top of the brainstem (see figure 3). In an evolutionary sense, the limbic system is one of the oldest of the brain's components. In fact, it used to be referred to as the old mammalian brain because it first appeared in the evolution of mammals. I refer to this portion of the brain as a system because it includes a vast array of interconnecting functions. The most basic survival instincts, including eating, procreating, fleeing from danger, physical protection, and fighting off

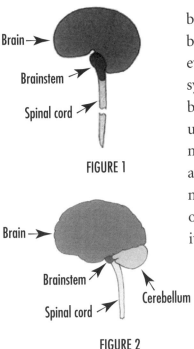

Brain→

Brainstem

Spinal cord

FIGURE 1

Brain→

Brainstem

Spinal cord

Cerebellum

FIGURE 2

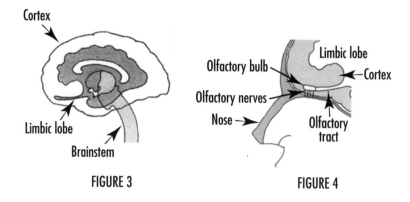

FIGURE 3   FIGURE 4

attackers, comprise a realm controlled by the limbic brain. The limbic system also rules over emotions, which is why the limbic brain is sometimes called the emotional brain. Look at your limbic system as the source of pleasure and discomfort, both of which can propel you to take action.

The limbic brain surrounds and is directly linked to the *olfactory bulb,* which processes odor signals (see figure 4). Olfaction, our sense of smell, is the only sense with a direct link to the emotions and our basic instincts. When you catch a whiff of your lover's perfume and your mood lifts and then you begin to think about sex, that is your brain responding to the remembered odor. When you smell the odor of freshly baked bread, you may begin to think about a parent or grandparent whose kitchen always smelled of baking bread, which may trigger a wave of nostalgia over that long-gone time in your life. You may also start thinking about how good a piece of fresh bread would taste and you may start to crave bread or similar foods. This momentary craving does not mean you are weak, or if you are trying to shed a few pounds that you lack determination. The craving is simply an impulse and often passes as quickly as it appears. Your response tells you that your sense of smell and the limbic brain are operating exactly as they are supposed to. Our early ancestors needed the sense of smell to lead them to sources of food and to alert them to the presence of predators. Modern culture has tended to minimize the importance of the sense of smell, primarily because it is not as well understood as the other senses and is linked to the so-called lower functions.

Hippocampus

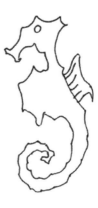

The hippocampus is an essential part of the limbic system (see figure 5), so essential we have two hippocampi, one on each side of the limbic brain and located above the ear about an inch and a half inside the skull. The term *hippocampus* is derived from the Latin name for seahorse, because early anatomists thought that it resembled the curling tail of a seahorse.

The *hippocampi* act as master librarians of information. They catalog, index, and direct information to its appropriate storage area. As you will see, the hippocampus has a complex

FIGURE 5

and elaborate part to play in various types of memory, and damage to this part of the brain can adversely affect memory and the day-to-day functions that require certain kinds of memory. Other important components of the limbic brain are the *mammillary* bodies, so named because they resemble tiny breasts.

Just above the nose, two important regulatory structures, the *hypothalamus* and the *pituitary*, bring us into the hormonal realm. The communication between the hypothalamus and the pituitary depends on and signals hormonal production.

The almond-shaped *amygdala* is another component of the limbic system and is essential for activating aggression and strong emotional responses and memory (see figure 6). When the amygdala stimulates the hippocampus, it is saying, "Wake up—this is important," and our attention is focused on the

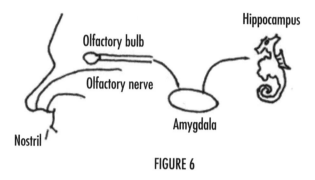

FIGURE 6

strong stimulus. The olfactory system is essential here because odors project through the amygdala, which then activates the hippocampi. So, if an odor triggers a strong nostalgic response, the amygdala has activated the hippocampi, which "directs" the retrieval of the memory from the *neocortex*, or higher conscious brain. This process is difficult to adequately explain because it is happening continually and so rapidly we aren't conscious of the individual steps. That, too, is the beauty of the system. We do not need to think about it or coax it into action.

Looked at as a whole, the limbic system allows us to use intellectual centers of the brain without concerning ourselves with breathing, keeping our heart beating, digesting our food, regulating our body temperature or blood pressure, or any of the other basic physical functions we take for granted. The limbic system hums along, monitoring and regulating a variety of functions, and then in an instant its powerful functions can swing into "high gear." If we smell smoke in the house and must jump out of bed and break down doors to alert the children, it is the limbic system that stimulates the reticular activating system to awaken us. The limbic brain controls "fight or flight" actions, often taken without conscious reasoning. Through a complex series of chemical responses, we have stamina and strength we didn't know we had. Meanwhile, the limbic system stimulates both profound fear and relief, as well as violent rage and tender love. The limbic system allows us to enjoy the range of emotions from mild to intense, and it provides information about what is important to us. We are most likely to pay attention to a learning task if our emotions help us perceive and define its larger meaning in our lives.

Moving Up to the Higher Functions

The largest portion of the brain, the *cerebrum*, covers the limbic brain like a cap. The cerebrum has two parts, which we refer to as the right and left brain, although they are not equal in size—the left brain is wider than the right brain and is considered the dominant brain. These two halves do not work strictly independently, but rather are connected by the *corpus callosum*, which is a thick network of nerve fibers—about 300 million of them. The two sides of the body act in a coordinated way and function as a whole because of this complex communication system between the two sides of the brain.

Each side of the brain is responsible for a variety of functions. The left brain is associated with logic, reasoning, language, and the ability to do mathematical calculations. The right brain is involved with our visual-spatial functions and music. We also associate creativity with the right brain. As I will discuss in detail later, the two sides of the brain can be activated—stimulated—through the olfactory system, which has implications for using odors to enhance learning and memory.

About 70 percent of our brain cells are found on the surface of the cerebrum, the *cerebral cortex*, which means "rind" or "bark" in Latin. In popular language, we call it "gray matter," even though its color has a pinkish cast.

The Busy Cerebrum

Each side of the cerebrum has four different *lobes* (see figure 7). The *occipital lobes*, located at the back of the head, are home for the *visual cortex*. The *parietal* lobes arch over the top of the head and contain the maps— or detailed schematics—corresponding to parts and sensations of the body.

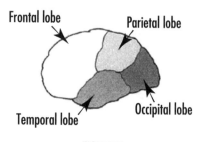

Frontal lobe Parietal lobe

Temporal lobe Occipital lobe

FIGURE 7

In evolutionary development, the *frontal* lobes, just behind the forehead, are the most recent addition to the human brain and are also the biggest lobes. The frontal cortex is almost 30 percent of the brain surface in humans, as compared to about 17 percent in our evolutionary cousin, the chimpanzee. The frontal lobes are critical to human behavior and function. Unlike other animals, we can plan what we will do in the next five minutes or the next five years. The frontal lobes allow us to do this. If the plan doesn't work, the frontal lobes allow us to figure out a new one.

One of the most controversial surgical procedures ever developed is the *prefrontal lobotomy*. It involves cutting nerve fibers in the forward portion of the frontal cortex. The nerve fibers involved are those that connect the prefrontal cortex to the rest of the brain. Damaging this portion of the brain essentially removes an individual's personality characteristics and usually promotes a passive, apathetic demeanor. This surgical procedure was developed as a treatment for mentally ill patients who did not respond to other therapies and as a drastic treatment for severe epilepsy. The profound change in behavior that can occur when a frontal lobe lobotomy is performed was dramatically depicted in the book, *One Flew Over the Cuckoo's*

Nest, by Ken Kesey, and of course in the movie by the same name. The ethics involved in removing an individual's defining personality characteristics for the sake of controlling his or her behavior remain in question.

The surgery itself was always considered highly experimental and controversial. In part, it became an idea considered worthy of experimentation because of data gathered from observing a patient who had a tragic—and bizarre—accident. The patient was Phineas Gage, a young foreman on a railroad crew. In 1848, a worksite explosion caused a long iron rod to be propelled through Gage's cheek and up through his skull. What was most amazing about the accident was that Gage lived; he apparently never lost consciousness and after a two-month hospital stay he was released and considered normal, except for the rod that remained lodged in his skull.

What Gage did lose, however, was his ability to live normally in society. True, he could speak, his memory was intact, and he was apparently still intellectually sharp. But he lost judgment, the ability to make a decision about the future and act on it, his sense of responsibility, and his social skills. For example, Gage was unable to discern when it was okay to use profane language (presumably with his male cohorts) and when the same language was unacceptable (probably when "ladies" were present). Once an aggressive worker interested in getting ahead, Gage lost his ambition and drive.

After some years of drifting from job to job, and even a short stint with P.T. Barnum's Circus in New York, Gage died in California. Five years after he was buried—rod and all—his body was removed from the grave and his skull eventually ended up in a display case at the Harvard Medical College in Boston. This unfortunate man's experience led to the notion that if a personality change could happen by accident, a surgical procedure could be developed for the purpose of altering personality. The lobotomy was never a precise surgery and involved significant guesswork. For the most part, it has fallen out of favor, replaced by less invasive drug therapies.

Moving On to the Temporal Lobes

Located on each side of the head, just above the ears, the *temporal* lobes are also important for self-concept and personality development. The *auditory cortex,* where sound is processed, is located in the temporal lobe. The temporal lobe is also essential for memory, particularly for transferring data from short-term memory into long-term storage. The long-term storage of information is what gives us our unique life. As you will see, when the temporal lobe is seriously damaged it may become impossible to function normally because the past virtually disappears and newly acquired information is not really learned because it isn't stored. Names (even one's own name), faces, places, events, language, and so forth are not retained if the temporal lobes are not functioning.

On one level we can understand memory anatomically as a process whereby we recall sensory stimuli. We read or hear words and convert the words to images. The temporal lobe processes the sounds, and the occipital lobe processes the stimuli of words, written or spoken, into the images. These visual images serve as signals that are transmitted through the *circuit of Papez,* the anatomical pathway that allows emotions to be generated. The *memory engram*—a memory trace—travels through this circuit and winds its way through three essential brain structures. The hippocampi are essential for immediate and short-term retention and as head librarian of the brain, probably play a major role in organizing and categorizing information; mammillary bodies are important for visual memory and other aspects of short-term memory; the *ventromedial nucleus* of the *thalamus* is essential for short-term storage of the memory engram.

Trauma to the brain and diseases that affect different parts of the brain can have a profound effect on memory and learning, as well as on the basic structure of the personality. The brain is resilient, however, and is sometimes able to compensate for damage in one area by stimulating another area to take over its function.

Electrical and Chemical Networks

The brain structures could not function were it not for the complex and ever-changing electrical and chemical networks that communicate 24 hours a day. Information travels through *neurons,* which come in many shapes and sizes (see figure 8).

Each neuron has a *control center,* cell body, and an *axon,* which is the component that transmits information somewhat like a telephone: The phone represents the cell body and the telephone wires are like the axon. Small fibers extend from the axon and there is a tiny bulb at the end of each fiber. The bulb is known as the *synaptic button.* *Dendrites,* which are also fibers, extend from the body of the cell. The *synaptic cleft* is a gap

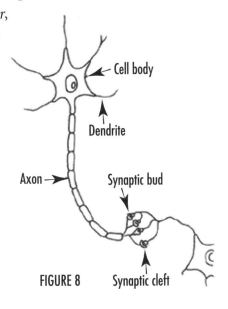

FIGURE 8

between the axon and the dendrite of the neighboring neuron. The cleft is critical because this gap accounts for the ability of neurons to communicate—connect—with each other, by way of chemicals in the brain. In other words, brain activity is both electrical and chemical, and the process is so complex that scientists began to understand it only in the last century. Much of the knowledge of brain circuitry and chemistry has been amassed in the last twenty-five years.

Neurotransmitters are a collective name given to a group of chemicals that traverse the synaptic cleft and are responsible for a variety of responses in the cells. Neurotransmitters involved in memory (among other functions) include *glutamate, acetylcholine, norepinephrine, serotonin,* and *dopamine.* Some brain chemicals have the ability to excite or activate brain activity; others dampen activity or quiet the brain. In addition, some of the neurotransmitters important for memory are also important in the olfactory system.

It is nearly impossible to view any activity of the brain one cell or one chemical at a time. Each of us has 100 billion neurons in our brain, a number that is difficult for most of us to "wrap our brain around." Neurons are sending and receiving messages constantly, and they can do more than one thing at a time. Much of what is continuously transmitted is involved in functions we are not consciously aware of most of the time. We do not think about making our eyes see, nor do we consciously monitor our hormone levels or direct enzymes to digest our food. When we sit down to type at a computer we make the decision to place our fingers on the keyboard, but once we start the activity we no longer need to think about directing each finger to strike the keys that form the words or number patterns we bring out of memory storage. Hundreds of bodily functions are occurring simultaneously and most of the time we don't give them—or the brain—much thought. When we can't remember a name or an event we may tap our head and demand that the brain get going and retrieve it for us. The awareness that we don't remember something is itself an intricate brain function!

It's All Like Floating Seaweed

Concepts about the brain and its capacities and mechanisms have changed over time. Just 25 years ago when I was in medical school, the brain was viewed as a static structure. A neuron, for example, was said to maintain its original structure and could not be changed. This turned out to be a limited concept, however. Research into brain cytolology revealed that the neuron is a dynamic system, ever changing and adapting. Imagine that the brain is like a vast ocean and the nerve cells within it are floating clumps of seaweed. Just as seaweed changes with ocean currents, the nerve cells in the brain add synapses or drop them. Synapses degenerate or increase in integrity, depending on stimulation and other factors in the environment. This process is going on constantly without our awareness. Just as an organism or a toxin in the ocean can damage or destroy the environment, a *neurotoxin* can come along and destroy neurons. This is why it is so important to protect the environment of the brain, just as we now realize how important it is to maintain and protect the biological environment of the planet.

It is natural to lose some neurons as we age. After age 18, we lose about 100,000 nerve cells a day and we can't change this. However, we can enhance the nature of the remaining nerve cells. They can adapt and change with us. Each cell resembles a bush with multiple twigs. A decline in our mental powers does not necessarily occur because we lose nerve cells. Absent injury or organic brain disease, we lose mental capacities because we do not stimulate nerve cells and hence, we do not add new "twigs" to the bush or maintain the integrity of the cells.

Throughout this book, you will find easy to implement tips and exercises designed to help you enhance brain function, learning, and memory. Just about any routine activities can serve as opportunities to stimulate nerve cells and sharpen your brain power in only a few minutes a day. Have fun with "The 7-Minute Shower Workout" (see page 52).

Feeding the Brain

It makes little sense to be concerned about your memory and ability to learn if you ignore the basics of brain care. For example, the brain requires about 20 percent of the body's oxygen, and such things as cigarette smoking and exposure to carbon monoxide compromise the oxygen supply to the brain. Research has demonstrated that even low-level exposure to carbon monoxide can result in impairment of such functions as memory, learning, concentration, abstract thinking, and visual-spatial skills.

We usually associate carbon monoxide with auto emissions, but kerosene heaters are for some individuals a continuous source of high concentrations of carbon monoxide. It is very important to keep all kerosene heaters and stoves, even the most recent models, only in a well-ventilated space. Even if you use a kerosene heater only for emergency heat during electrical power outages, you risk exposure to low levels of carbon monoxide during the hours it is in use. Extreme caution is necessary when using these heaters, and camp stoves and kerosene boat heaters and stoves must also be used with care.

The brain also guzzles calories; the brain uses 30 percent of your daily intake of calories. The brain requires a steady diet of glucose (blood sugar), and if it doesn't get it you may feel sluggish and your mental abilities may become impaired. Many people skip breakfast, but this is a bad idea because blood sugar levels are low after a night's sleep. A study of British college students showed that those who ate breakfast performed better on memory tests than those who skipped the breakfast. Consuming five or six small meals, or three meals and two or three snacks, keeps blood sugar levels even throughout the day. Ideally, your meals and snacks should contain each of the macronutrients: protein, carbohydrates, and a small amount of fat.

Can Dieting Be Detrimental to Your Memory?

Individuals who are on diets must be careful not to drop below a minimum of 1200 calories a day. If they do, they risk depriving the brain of the fuel it needs to operate efficiently. A study conducted at the Institute of Food Research in Reading, England, found that women on a low-calorie diet of below 1,200 calories a day had impaired reaction time and concentration, as well as difficulties with immediate memory, when compared to women consuming a moderate amount of calories. This is just one more reason to avoid any form of extreme dieting.

Have A Power Lunch—Reach For the Protein

The amino acids tyrosine and tryptophan have a special role in influencing neurotransmitter production. Specifically, the brain uses tyrosine to produce dopamine and norepinephrine, which promote an alert and awake state, quick and sharp thinking, memory, and fast reactions. Tryptophan influences serotonin production, which promotes a more relaxed, unfocused state that can interfere with concentration.

The two amino acids compete with one another, which means that the type of meal you eat will determine which neurotransmitter will dominate. According to researcher Judith Wurtman, Ph.D., of M.I.T., you can manipulate your mental state with your diet and even with the order in which you eat the various foods in a meal. For example, if you want to promote mental sharpness, Dr. Wurtman recommends eating protein foods before you eat the carbohydrates because the tyrosine in the protein will reach the brain first and trigger the production of dopamine and norepinephrine.

If you take this advice, a true "power lunch" would be some protein foods such as poultry or fish, followed by a green salad and some fruit. If you order a chicken salad sandwich, for example, take the chicken off the bread and eat it the protein first. This should boost your mental energy in the afternoon. If you want to relax in the evening, then eat the carbohydrate foods first. The serotonin produced will help you wind down. If you experience sleepiness after lunch or dinner, try manipulating the order in which you eat your foods and monitoring how alert you feel.

As a "brain-booster," tyrosine appears to be very powerful and may modulate the effects of stress. The U.S. Army Research Institute of Environmental Medicine tested tyrosine on soldiers under stressful conditions. The soldiers, ages 18 to 20, experienced a simulated sudden airlift of over 15,000 feet, with the added stress of a cold temperature. The simulation was done twice, each session lasting 4½ hours. Before the simulations, the soldiers were given either tyrosine or a placebo. During the simulation the soldiers were tested for clear thinking and performed tasks requiring concentration. The results showed that tyrosine diminished the stress among those soldiers who found the situation stressful in the first place. But the tyrosine did not affect those who didn't find the simulation exercise particularly stressful. So, if you anticipate a stressful event, eating a high-protein meal may modulate your response to the stress and enable you to think clearly.

Nourishing Your Brain Every Day

Your brain requires *20 percent* of your body's oxygen, so:

+ Do not smoke or expose yourself to secondhand smoke.

+ Avoid exposure to carbon monoxide—beware of
auto emissions and carbon monoxide leaks from
kerosene camp stoves and heaters. If you use these
products during power outages or for camping or
boating, check the ventilation. Never use these items
when you sleep.

+ Fireplaces and woodstoves suck oxygen from a room.
Make sure they are working properly—smoke should
not back up into the room.

+ Invest in a carbon monoxide detector.

Your brain consumes *30 percent* of the calories you take in
every day, so:

+ Never consume fewer than 1,200 calories a day.

+ Always eat breakfast—don't deprive your brain of
needed energy.

+ Small frequent meals help the brain maintain a
steady supply of glucose better than one or two large
meals do.

+ All meals and snacks should have protein, carbohydrates, and a small amount of fat.

The Great Amino Acid Race

The "raw materials" of brain power:

Protein foods contain the *amino acid tyrosine* and the brain
uses tyrosine to produce the neurotransmitters *dopamine* and
norepinephrine, which in turn promote an alert and awake
state. If you want to be at your intellectual best, eat the protein
portion of your meal first and give the amino acids a head start

in the race to produce these neurotransmitters. Eat your scrambled eggs before you eat your toast and fruit; order salmon salad for lunch or don't reach for the basket of rolls until you've finished the salmon.

The "raw materials" of relaxation:

Many carbohydrate foods contain the *amino acid tryptophan* and the brain uses it to produce serotonin, which promotes relaxation. If you want to wind down, give tryptophan a head start and let serotonin dominate. So, go ahead and nibble on bread before you cut into the chicken breast. Eat your fried rice or vegetarian pasta meal for dinner and relax as the serotonin influence has the edge.

Experiment with these "food order" ideas and track how you feel. It's only the order of consumption that changes, not necessarily the composition of your meals. As mentioned, all meals and snacks should contain protein, carbohydrates, and a small amount of fat.

Caffeine—Yes or No?

Caffeine can promote a sharp mind, but it can also make you dull. One cup of a caffeinated drink such as coffee or tea can boost your thinking ability and the effect can last up to six hours, but overindulge in caffeine and your brain doesn't like it. In a study of college students in Britain, students were given 125 milligrams of caffeine (about the amount in one large cup or mug of coffee), 250 milligrams of caffeine, or no caffeine. The students then performed a battery of mental performance tests. Performance on most of the tests did not vary significantly among the three groups of students. However, on a numerical test the group given the largest dose of caffeine made the most mistakes. The group that was not under the influence of any caffeine did the best, with the 125-milligram group falling in between.

It appears that caffeine can interfere with performance of certain kinds of tasks. Unless you need to do calculations quickly, one to two cups of coffee or tea may help you feel alert and keep your thinking clear. But go for a third or fourth cup and the added caffeine is likely to interfere with focused concentration.

Nutrients for the Brain

You need a wide range of *micronutrients*, or vitamins and minerals, every day, so it is never wise to isolate nutrients and emphasize them at the expense of the others. However, the B vitamins, particularly B6, have functions in the body that affect mental state in specific ways. Tryptophan, the amino acid that promotes relaxation, needs B6 to work. The recommended daily allowance (RDA) is 1.6 milligrams for men, but it is likely that *both men and women need 20 milligrams* for optimal function. (20 milligrams is well within the range of a safe dose of vitamin B6.) Thiamine (B1), riboflavin (B2), niacin (B3), B12, and folic acid are also essential for mental functioning. The RDAs of these vitamins also tend to be lower than what is optimal, which is why many physicians and nutritionists recommend taking a vitamin supplement. I recommend that you discuss taking an appropriate multivitamin supplement with your physician. Taking dietary supplements does not mean that you can be careless with your diet, however. The various B vitamins are liberally found in the basic food groups: grains, fruits, vegetables, beans and legumes, and dairy products and other animal protein.

Like vitamins, minerals are important for optimal brain function. Iron, for example, carries oxygen in the body, making adequate iron necessary for oxygen to reach the brain.

Inadequate iron levels, as indicated by low hemoglobin levels, have been shown to interfere with work productivity. Inadequate copper, boron, and manganese can lead to impaired memory and mood. The minerals copper and zinc compete with one another in the body, and it appears that when zinc is dominant, it promotes a depressed or anxious mood. Copper, which is found in seafood and fruits and vegetables, promotes more positive mood states, so it is important to eat these foods to balance zinc levels, especially if you enjoy oysters or organ meats, which contain generous amounts of zinc.

The Antioxidants—An Orange and a Carrot a Day Keep the Doctor Away

Antioxidant nutrients are significant in preventing and even reversing some diseases and conditions. The primary job of antioxidants is preventing damage to the body caused by *free radicals*, which are unstable and reactive molecules. Normal metabolic processes produce free radicals and vigorous exercise can produce them too. But exposure to toxic chemicals or radiation, for example, also creates an environment for free radical production. Fortunately, the body has a group of enzymes, collectively known as free radical scavengers, whose job is to neutralize free radicals and prevent damage.

Vitamins C and E, beta carotene, and the mineral selenium are powerful antioxidant nutrients because they protect the body from the damage caused by free radicals. This is a relatively new area of preventive medicine, but information about the benefits of antioxidant nutrients is rapidly accumulating. Antioxidants may prevent and help reverse heart disease and may play a role in preventing cancer by strengthening the immune system. Their value extends to preventing common infections and enhancing brain function. For example, preliminary research suggests that vitamin E may play a role in slowing the progression of Alzheimer's disease, and vitamin C may, among other benefits, boost memory, especially in the elderly. A 1997 survey conducted in Spain found a correlation between high scores on mental function tests and consumption of generous amounts of fruits, vegetables, and fiber. Beta carotene, another powerful antioxidant, is found in fruits and vegetables and in abundant concentrations in those that are yellow and orange. Given what we already know about antioxidants, eating an orange and a carrot a day—along with the proverbial apple—may indeed help keep the doctor away.

The Memory Tree

You have probably heard advertisements for *ginkgo biloba*, which is an ornamental tree. The leaves of this tree have properties that appear to improve memory, and they appear to have positive effects on blood circulation as well as on brain function. In Germany and France, it is prescribed as a treatment to improve mental functioning in the elderly and for senile dementia and Alzheimer's disease. These claims are backed up by scientific studies, most conducted in Germany.

Ginkgo is a powerful antioxidant, and it is believed that it helps maintain the integrity of neurons, as well as improving blood flow to the brain. It is generally recommended that one begin taking ginkgo when problems with memory first appear and are mild. Recommended dosages vary from 120 milligrams a day, divided into three doses, for mild memory impairment to 240 milligrams a day as a treatment for serious dementia and Alzheimer's disease. Its effectiveness remains controversial. An article in the *Journal of the American Medical Association* from the summer of 2002 found that gingko was no more efficient than sugar pills in improving memory. I do not believe you

39

should self-medicate with ginkgo, but should talk with your doctor before taking this medicinal plant. While it appears safe, it should be taken under supervision.

The Nose Enters the Picture

There is a strong overlap between the anatomic and neuro-chemical structures for olfaction and for memory. Even if we did not know the scientific reasons behind the connections, we can observe them in a clinical setting. For example, trauma to the head often results in loss or diminishment of the sense of smell and sometimes in temporary memory lapses. (Amnesia, a more severe disturbance in memory, will be discussed later.)

When I was a medical student at the University of Michigan, I rode a bicycle around the campus, and one November after-noon, when I was on the way to my surgical rotation at the VA hospital I was hit by a car, thrown off my bike, and knocked out. (This was before the days that bicyclists wore the sensible hel-mets that most people use today—I highly recommend them.) I spent some time in the hospital, and then for several months after the accident everything smelled like cigarette smoke, although I wasn't a smoker. I also had difficulty recalling words—not all words, of course, but certain words and terms, some of which were important to clinical work in which I was involved. For example, two weeks after being discharged from the hospital I couldn't think of the term "blood bank." Eventually, however, both my memory and my sense of smell returned to normal.

My experience is quite typical of what we see in many patients with head trauma. They may lose their sense of smell altogether or experience "phantom" smells as I did. Different parts of the memory may be temporarily disturbed. When the head trauma heals, the sense of smell usually comes back and memory returns to normal.

Odor Molecules and the Brain

The best way to illustrate how olfaction works, and how it is connected to memory, is to follow the path of an odor molecule from the air to recognition in the brain. It all starts with taking a breath. When we inhale, the odor molecules move up through the nose and eventually reach the *epithelial lining* of the top of the nose and from there they reach a pin-sized area where the *olfactory nerves* are located.

It sounds paradoxical, but when the nose is somewhat stuffy, more odor molecules reach the epithelium. When the nose is partially stuffed up, air currents—little tornadoes—form, which act like a trap, giving the molecules an opportunity to reach the epithelium. Just as the body has many cycles, such as the sleep/wakefulness cycle or the menstrual cycle, there is also an olfactory cycle. In the olfactory cycle, one nostril is more stuffed up or closed and the other is open. It is through this stuffed-up nostril that most odor molecules reach the epithelium. This is the nostril that has the better olfactory accuracy during this phase of the olfactory cycle. Every four to eight hours the olfactory cycle changes; the previously open nostril is more closed, and the closed nostril opens. We could look at this cycle as having an active and a resting phase. Every few hours the resting nostril becomes active and the previously active nostril rests.

You can experience the olfactory cycle for yourself. Simply put your thumb or a finger against one side of your nose to close that nostril. When you inhale you will perceive that the nostril is open or stuffy. Now close the other nostril and inhale again. You will be able to tell the difference between the amount of air you can inhale in each nostril. The nostril that is more stuffed up is the nostril through which most of the odor molecules will reach the olfactory nerves. If you have a bad cold, however, and you are unable to breathe through your nose at all, this principle does not operate and your sense of smell is diminished.

Changing the Olfactory Cycle

The olfactory cycle changes naturally on its own and most people are unaware that they even have such a cycle going on. Most of the time the olfactory cycle is inconsequential. However, when looking at memory in relation to left-brain/right-brain functions, we can actually activate one side of the brain by changing the olfactory cycle (see page 54).

The Molecule Keeps Traveling

Once they are up in the nose, the odor molecules reach the olfactory epithelia, the smell center located just behind the bridge of the nose. The epithelia are mucous-coated membranes about the size of a dime. As the odor molecules move through the thin membrane, they reach a pin-sized area where millions of receptor sites are located. These receptor sites allow us to distinguish between odors and identify them. Distinguishing and identifying different odors is, of course, something we learn and remember.

The body's electrical system is involved because neurons fire off as an indication that a particular odorant is present. The odor signal travels through the *cribriform plate*, a paper-thin part of the skull through which olfactory nerves are projected from tiny holes. (The word "cribriform" means "pierced with small holes.") When the odor molecule reaches the olfactory bulb, which is in the brain itself, it is intensified by a factor of about 1,000. In other words, the brain intensifies and transforms the molecule a thousand times in order to respond to the odor. Obviously this process happens so rapidly that we do not experience it step by step, nor are we conscious of it. The mechanism by which an odor is intensified is what allows us to detect about 10,000 different odors.

Glandular secretions in the nose keep it moist. Moist conditions, including breathing in moist air, promote better ability to smell and allow a greater quantity of odor molecules to be absorbed. If you are walking in the woods after a warm summer rain, the earthy scents seem to be stronger, but it is the moist warm air that is allowing you to inhale more of the rich odors of the soil and trees.

We also smell more efficiently if we breathe through the nose because it appears that the brain is more sensitive to smells through nasal breathing. Comparison of brainwave activity also indicates that we are more alert when we inhale through the nose. If you are exercising vigorously, for example, and begin to breathe through your mouth, your ability to detect the odors around you will diminish. The same thing happens when you have a cold and your food is tasteless because you are unable to smell it.

Learning and Memory Tip

Nasal breathing can act like a substitute for coffee. If you are feeling drowsy or have difficulty concentrating on a task, take deep breaths through your nose—your will stimulate the brain waves that promote an alert state. Caffeine can lead to alertness but it produces other effects on the body when consumed in excess. So, when you first start experiencing an energy drop or are having trouble focusing, stop breathing through your mouth and start breathing through your nose. This is probably the easiest learning and memory tip and can be used by everyone.

In addition to the olfactory apparatus, we have a nerve called the *trigeminal nerve*, which is the part of the nervous system that allows us to feel sensations on the face. If your eyes water when you peel an onion, it is because the trigeminal nerve has been irritated. Even those who have for the most part lost their sense of smell will react to the strong smell of ammonia in smelling salts. The trigeminal nerve allows that response to occur.

The ability to smell is not uniform among species. Dogs, for example, can detect some odors ten million times better than humans. The tooth whale is anosmic, meaning it has no sense of smell at all. Among normal humans, one person's ability to detect certain odors, such as orange, may be 4,000 times better than another person's ability to detect the same smell. So, your spouse's ability to smell the garbage under the sink may be much better than yours. In general, women have a better sense of smell than men; among women of reproductive age, this ability increases during the time of ovulation.

The sense of smell is unique among the senses in that its pathway to the brain is direct. The other senses have processing structures that block their direct route to the brain. For example, the ear has the eardrum that functions as a barrier outside the brain between the auditory processing system and sound. The eye has the cornea, which acts as a barrier between visual stimuli and the visual processing system. The nose, however, is a direct, unencumbered pathway to the brain, and the olfactory bulb is part of the limbic brain, the seat of emotions.

React First, Identify Later

More than any other sense, the sense of smell is "irrational." Sensory stimuli from the other senses are processed first in the *thalamus*. The thalamus is the part of the brain that acts as a relay point between the sensory organs and the cerebral cortex, the cognitive center of the brain. This pathway is what enables us to identify stimuli before we evaluate or judge it. The sense of smell works in the reverse. When we detect an odor in the air, we decide if we like it before we identify it. If I show you a picture of a tree, you will identify it as a tree before you decide if you like it. If I place the odor of pine under your nose, you will react positively or negatively to the odor before you identify it as pine.

When you detect an odor in the air that affects you emotionally, it may take a few seconds to understand why you are sad or happy or perhaps distressed or disturbed in some way. You may even be overcome with a wave of nostalgia, which is usually a bittersweet response. The limbic brain has gone to work before your rational brain knows why you are reacting. That is what makes the sense of smell seem so irrational. You can be going about your business one minute and close to tears the next all because of an odor. It doesn't make sense, you say, and you're right. It doesn't make sense because nature designed the olfactory system to activate the emotions and survival instincts.

The fact that our sense of smell is linked to powerful emotions and survival instincts makes good evolutionary sense. Early humans had to be able to detect the presence of an animal, which could mean dinner or danger, before they could see it. Our ancient ancestors could probably "sniff out" the presence of edible plants far better than any of us can today.

You may think that act of yawning is a sign of distraction, even boredom, as well as sleepiness. It is possible that yawning is a remnant from our evolutionary past in which the ability to detect odors was integral to survival. Yawning brings in a large volume of air into your mouth and nose, thereby increasing the

odor molecules that reach the olfactory bulb. In our evolutionary past, yawning may have been one way to "sniff" the air for
predators before sleeping. This may sound far-fetched to our
modern ears, but consider that we find increased incidence of
generalized anxiety disorder among individuals with diminished
sense of smell. It is possible that this anxiety results in part
from an inability to feel safe because these individuals cannot
detect odors and therefore establish a sense of personal safety
within their environment. The mechanism of smell hasn't
changed just because we no longer need to sniff the air for lions
and tigers; the basic survival instinct remains and we are just
beginning to understand why loss of the ability to smell may be
linked to certain psychological disorders.

In Western culture, the nose has often been considered the
least important of the senses, in part because it is linked so
closely with emotional life, which is undervalued in our culture
precisely because it isn't "rational." In addition, our religious
traditions tend to label most things as either good or bad, and
the senses have been viewed with suspicion. After all, they may
lead us astray and off the path of "good" behavior. Naturally,
the most "emotional" of the senses has been regarded as a
prime suspect.

Western intellectuals have had their own reasons for encouraging dismissal of the importance of smell. Sigmund Freud, the
father of psychoanalysis, viewed the sense of smell as important
for "primitive" society, but not for the so-called advanced
cultures, whose focus was intellectual achievement. (At least he
thought it should be.) Early anthropologists observed that the
societies they studied incorporated the sense of smell into all
their rituals in an uninhibited way, and they too concluded that
placing importance on the sense of smell was something that
cultures would "outgrow" as they advanced. Obviously, there

was significant cultural bias in these conclusions, and it was a mistake to put the senses on a hierarchy of importance anyway.

When I was in medical school, very little classroom or clinical time was devoted to studying the sense of smell or diagnosing and treating patients who complained of losing olfactory accuracy. The role of olfaction in health or its potential role in diagnosing or treating illness is still largely ignored in today's medical practices. Some physicians still do not understand how devastating and even hazardous it is to lose the ability to smell.

The lack of assessment of smell and taste among adult patients remains in a sad state, especially when one considers that more two million people at any given time suffer from olfactory impairment. Olfactory assessment is particularly needed among hospitalized patients, those on medications that can impair taste and smell, and patients with neurological diseases and disorders such as Alzheimer's disease, Parkinson's disease, or stroke. Diminished ability to smell may be an early symptoms of Alzheimer's disease and olfactory testing may help separate different types of Parkinson's disease, some of which produce olfactory impairment and some of which do not. In addition, diminished ability to smell is associated with several psychiatric disorders including depression and generalized anxiety disorder, both of which influence memory. It is well worth the physician's time to perform simple screening tests for olfactory ability.

Recently, our foundation reviewed 94 physical examinations performed on patients at a major teaching hospital in Chicago. These patients could respond verbally and suffered from conditions in which one could anticipate diminished ability to smell. In none of these examinations was olfactory testing performed. Since most people do not realize that their ability to smell is impaired, we cannot count on patients to report this symptom.

In fact, many patients would not necessarily consider loss of smell a symptom at all. If screening tests for olfactory ability are not part of physical examinations in a prominent teaching hospital in a major metropolitan area, it is unlikely that they are performed in small community hospitals throughout the country.

In our clinic, I have listened to people talk about how isolated they feel when they can't enjoy the aroma of food or when they look at flowers but can't smell any fragrance. Without a sense of smell, life loses an important dimension and often seems flat or as if something significant is missing. More than any other sense, we take it for granted until it is gone. Losing the ability to smell also has serious implications for survival. Individuals who lack the ability to smell are at risk because they are unable to detect gas leaks or smoke, and the instinct to escape toxic fumes before they cause harm is compromised. Some individuals who lose their ability to smell become socially isolated because they are insecure about how *they* smell. They become anxious and begin to interpret any social rejection as a reaction to how they smell.

The sense of smell, however, has made a comeback in the last decade or so. Some recent medical research has focused on the physiology of the olfactory system; other research has studied the way odors influence behavior, including consumer behavior, social interaction, and sexuality. As you are no doubt aware, the pleasant aromas in the shopping mall are not accidental. We and other researchers have determined which odors influence shoppers to spend more money in retail stores, and research into the commercial use of odors is vast and ongoing in the United States, Europe, and Japan. Odors that influence both male and female sexual arousal have also been the subject of research at The Smell and Taste Treatment and Research

Foundation and others have entered this research area too. The scents of pumpkin pie and lavender were the "top-performing" odors in our study that increased arousal in men; the odor of cucumber and Good & Plenty candy were the two "winning" odors in our female arousal study.

The Language of Smell

Olfaction has its own language:

Anosmia, the lack of ability to smell.

Hyposmia, diminished ability to smell.

Phantosmia, hallucinated smell, often unpleasant in nature. This is particularly difficult to deal with because the person may believe that he or she smells bad and others can detect that this foul smell is coming from them.

Dysosmia, a situation in which something does not smell the way it should.

Malodor, an unpleasant or even potentially toxic odor in the environment. Malodors are an important issue because unpleasant odors in the environment can impair learning and memory. Unpleasant odors can even increase aggression, which has implications for many settings, including schools and places of work.

Hyperosmia, a greatly increased ability to smell, which can cause unique problems. For example, we once tested a woman whose sense of smell was so sensitive that she could smell much better than the average dog. Our patient was miserable. She was unable to shop at malls or grocery stores because she was overwhelmed by the odors. She could not tolerate the artificial fragrances added to shampoos and other cosmetic products. Eventually it was discovered that this patient's hyperosmia was the result of Addison's disease, which affects the adrenal glands. She serves as an example of how difficult life can be when a sensory ability is greater than normal.

Taste Is Largely Dependent on Smell

Most people are unaware that about 90 percent of taste (*gustation*) is actually smell. We taste foods because we can smell them. One reason food why tastes so flat when you have a severe cold is that you can't smell it. If you hold your nose while you eat a piece of rich dark chocolate, it will taste like cardboard. An apple and an onion, or a potato and a carrot, all taste the same, and when the nose is blocked, coffee loses its strong aroma and flavor. When patients seek help because they believe they have lost their sense of taste, we test them for loss of ability to smell.

Gustation also has its own language:

Ageusia, lack of ability to taste.

Hypogeusia, reduced ability to taste.

Hypergeusia, the increased ability to taste.

Phantogeusia, phantom taste. Individuals who experience phantogeusia may become socially isolated because they worry about having bad breath; they may use mouthwash excessively or constantly chew on mints.

At any given time, *between 2 and 4 million people* in the United States suffer from temporary or permanent impairments of smell and taste. We are currently conducting research into effective treatments to restore the sense of smell in those who have lost it.

Odor Memory

Odors tend to be familiar after the first time we detect them. We may not be able to identify the odor, but we recognize it as an odor we have experienced before. Recognition of an odor is not the same as identifying it. For example, if you see a raspberry at the same time you are presented with the odor, it is easier to identify the smell. Odors are not remembered in fragments.

You may recognize a familiar face if you see just the eye or the nose, but odors are remembered as a whole, an overall impression. We may be able to identify a discrete odor within a mixture, but this is an area in which humans are not particularly proficient.

We also store odors unconsciously, meaning that we make no effort to retain the memory of an odor. The language of odor is problematic because it is difficult to describe what an odor smells like other than naming what produces the odor. A banana smells like a banana, pine trees smell like pine trees. We can describe the intensity of an odor and we can try to categorize the odors as sour or sweet or pungent. As you can see, these are words used to describe tastes. For the most part, however, smells tend to be described in terms of emotional evaluation: pleasant or unpleasant, bad or good. A smell may also be described by the way it causes one to feel: alert and bright or relaxed and content. Because olfaction and emotion are so closely linked it is not surprising that words such as euphoric, sickening, uplifting, centered, passionate, or calm are used to describe responses to odors. An elderly woman once said that the smell of peppermint made her feel so energized and daring that she couldn't be held responsible for her actions after a few whiffs.

Odors, Memory, and Learning

The relationship between odors and memory and learning has also aroused interest, and as it turns out, it is a multifaceted relationship. The role of the sense of smell has in improving memory and learning, as well as in retrieval of information, is complex and involves tapping into what we know about (1) smell and the brain and (2) smell and emotional states. For example, odors have the power to influence mood, which in turn influences memory. Odors introduced into a learning environment can actually help us retain and retrieve information by first altering our mood or our sense of alertness or relaxation. In order to fully absorb the relationship between smell and memory, it is important to understand the various types of memory and learning, the subject of the next chapter.

The 7-Minute Shower Workout

You can begin to increase your brainpower by performing this mental exercise just seven minutes a day. Why seven minutes? The average shower lasts about seven minutes, so I recommend that you devote those few minutes to a mental workout. As you scrub yourself with your favorite scented soap, try these activities.

Name all the animals that begin with the letter A, then B, and so on through the alphabet. Or, name all the cities, book titles, or movies that begin with each letter.

Devise your own "brain teasers" by choosing a word of six letters or more and then think of all the words you can make from the letters. Try these: tragicomedy, brontosaurus, supercilious, and aardvark.

Do some calculations in your head. Figure percentages, visualize a column of numbers and add them without benefit of paper and pencil, then multiply them, and when you have that figure, divide it by three—or multiples of three. If you grew up in the age of calculators, recite all the multiplication tables—and resolve not to rely on a calculator for simple computations, such as figuring 15 and 20 percent tips!

Think geographically—test your knowledge of places and landmarks. What states border the Mississippi River? How many state capitals can you name? Visualize a map of Europe or Africa and take a mental trip through these continents as you name the countries. If you get stuck, look at an atlas later when you have a minute. The next day, do the exercise again to see how much you've learned.

Pick a year—any year—and try to remember as much as you can about it. Notice the associations you make and the cues you use to recall additional information. For example, think about the year you were eleven years old. What comes to mind first? Your teacher? Your best friend? Your home? A national or global event? If you do this exercise regularly, record your memories in a journal and eventually you'll have a mini-version of your life story.

If you enjoy reading fiction, plot a novel and develop the characters. What do they look like? How do they smell? What kind of trouble are they in and how will they get out of it? Where does the novel take place? In just seven minutes a day, you can develop an ongoing story.

Make your shower a feast for the senses:

Concentrate on the odor of the soap, the shampoo, the faint odor of chlorine in the water.

Listen to the sound of the water rushing through the shower-head and the variety of sounds the water produces as it flows off your body and splashes in the bathtub.

Feel the texture of the washcloth or sponge. How does the soap feel on your skin? How does the water feel as it hits your shoulders and back, your neck and face, and your arms and hands? Notice the sensation when you massage shampoo into your hair.

When your eyes are open, what do you see? Pay attention to the colors around you.

When you step out of the shower, concentrate on the odor of the towel you wrap around your body or the texture of the mat beneath your feet. Pay attention to the temperature change and the way the cooler air feels on your skin.

Note: If you shower with your partner, so much the better. Challenge each other. Play the word games together or test each other's knowledge of geography or history. Avoid getting too serious—keep the games fun and light.

Fun with the Left and Right Brain

You can enlist the olfactory cycle to help you activate the part of the brain you use for different types of activities. For example, let's say you want to activate the *left brain* in order to learn mathematics, language, or any activity that involves logical thinking. You will change the olfactory cycle by opening the *right* nostril, which means you want to close off the left nostril. So, press hard on your *left palm with the thumb on your right hand.*

If you want to activate the *right brain* in order to engage in a creative activity such as drawing or listening to music, then you want to open the *left nostril.* You can change the olfactory cycle by pressing hard on your *right palm with the thumb on your left hand.*

You will see from this experiment that you cannot look at physiological processes in isolation. Your changing olfactory cycle even influences the way you perform a variety of activities in your daily life.

Test Your Own Nose

This is the "alcohol sniff test," and you can perform it in your home. First, put some rubbing alcohol on a piece of cotton—a simple cotton ball is fine. Hold it underneath your chin and slightly away from your body. If you can smell the alcohol, your sense of smell is probably fine. If not, you may have a degree of olfactory impairment, and I recommend asking your doctor about more extensive testing. This alcohol sniff test is quite reliable as a screening test and correlates with other olfactory tests.

3

Memory Comes in Many Varieties

"The horror of that moment," the king went on, "I shall
never never forget."
"You will, though," the Queen said, "if you don't make
a memorandum of it."

— Lewis Carroll, *Through the Looking-Glass*

Consider your memory as a collection—a storehouse—of all
that you know and have experienced, from the most distant
recollection of your childhood to what you ate for lunch
yesterday. Neuropsychologist Larry Squire offers a good working
definition of the closely related concepts of learning and
memory. "Learning," he says, "is the *process* of acquiring new
information, while memory refers to the *persistence* of learning
in a state that can be revealed at a later time."

Memories of experiences or events are seldom emotionally
neutral. In most cases you label or classify memories as good or
bad, depending on the emotional tone of the memories. One
person may remember a family reunion as a fabulous event,
while another may say that he would never choose this crazy
group for friends and will certainly never go to another reunion.
You also have a variety of memories—*scripts*—that allow you
to effortlessly perform everyday functions, and you have a
storehouse of facts you need to navigate through the world.

Scientists who have studied memory have devised a variety of
classifications that help us understand how the brain functions,

and by extension, how humans function. These classifications also help us determine how human culture developed. Language, music, dance, mathematics, painting, and the ability to construct grass huts and log cabins or steel and glass skyscrapers are all rooted in specific kinds of stored knowledge, which we call memory.

As you will see, certain aptitudes and talents that appear to be stronger in some people than in others are related to and even correspond to particular types of memory. This does not mean that these aptitudes are totally absent in others, but most of us have greater potential to excel in certain skill areas than in others. However, what we call a talent or aptitude is meaningless if it isn't developed, and practice will improve most of the skills involved in learning and memory.

Remembering Facts/Knowing How

One way to look at memory is as a group of operating systems. These systems are integrated with one another, but each has different functions. Two broad classifications are *declarative memory* and *procedural memory*, sometimes referred to as "knowing that" and "knowing how." Declarative memory includes general knowledge. For example, you know that Charles Dickens wrote *Oliver Twist*, and that California is on the West Coast. It also includes your personal memories. You remember that you were 36 when you had your first child and you can vividly recall the day this baby skipped off to kindergarten.

Procedural memory involves knowing how to perform tasks and functions. Your declarative memory allows you to identify a violin, but if you can play it, that knowledge is a function of procedural memory. Playing tennis, hitting a home run, performing the tango, and making a pot of coffee involve procedural memory.

Declarative memory is further broken down into *semantic memory*, which includes just the facts, and *episodic memory* that describes our recollection of personal experiences. Knowing that Bali is an island in Indonesia is a fact, part of your semantic memory, but your recollection of walking on the beach in Bali at sunset is an episodic memory. You know that a war took place in Vietnam, which is a semantic memory. If you were a soldier in that war, your experiences live on as episodic memories. Perhaps more than any other classification, episodic memories define you as an individual because they form your autobiography.

Semantic memory also gives us our ability to express ourselves. Every language is a symbolic system with structure and rules. Language allows us to gives form to the associations we make. If I say the word "house," your mind immediately begins processing the concept and you may think about cleaning house, the White House, buying a house, painting the house, your first house, and so on. Semantic memory also includes the way our language expresses past, present, and future time and the way we identify spatial relationships—near and far, under and over, on and off, and so forth.

Lexical Memory

The memory for language and words is called *lexical memory*. Some people have high aptitude for language. You can always spot these individuals because they consistently win word games. I have friends, the Cowens, who are expert Scrabble players. As a team, this couple is like a walking thesaurus. They write direct mail pieces for a living, but their avocation is language. I compare their superior vocabulary to that of William Shakespeare, who used more different words in his plays than any other writer. Generally, we perceive those who have good lexical memory as being more intelligent than others with more limited vocabulary because our culture places high value on language skills.

Lexical memory is recorded in the brain both visually and through the auditory system and is processed in the left hemisphere. As you know, written language developed much later than spoken language in human culture. Before written language appeared, those with superior lexical memory were no doubt the individuals chosen to carry the history of the society. If you saw the television miniseries *Roots*, author Alex Haley was able to trace his own family's genealogical roots by listening to a *griot*, a tribal historian, recite the names of men and women born into the African tribe from which he was descended. The griot had the ability to recall every birth in his tribe going back many hundreds of years. Some Native American groups have a similar oral tradition, through which genealogy and culture is passed. Clearly, only a person with superb lexical memory could be an oral historian, and since ancient times it has been considered a high-status position.

Plato was among the ancient philosophers who feared that written language would negatively affect the ability to remember. And it is true that the purported lexical memory of some of the ancients was remarkable. It is said that the Athenian Themistocles knew the name of each of the 20,000 citizens of Athens. Xerxes knew the names of all his 100,000 soldiers. Today, we read *The Iliad* and *The Odyssey*, but the 27,000 lines of Homer's epics were once recited. In medieval Europe, recitation contests were gala events, and the typical *jongleur*, or minstrel, could memorize an epic poem of hundreds of lines after hearing it only three times. Superior memorization skills seem impossible to many of us and are no longer necessary to function in society. But memorizing poetry, passages from sacred literature, or important speeches can be a valuable component of a mental workout. (See "Sharpen Your Ability to Memorize" on page 85.)

You know you have a lapse in lexical memory when you know a word but just can't call it up, so to speak. You may say, "It's on the tip of my tongue," because it feels that close to the surface. These words almost always come back once you have stopped thinking about the fact that you can't remember them.

Kinesthetic Memory

When you watch Tara Lipinski or Scott Hamilton glide across the ice and do their triple jumps and reverse camel spins, you are watching an example of *kinesthetic memory*. You have heard this referred to as "muscle memory," but it is really the brain that learns and remembers what the muscles require. It is easy to see why kinesthetic memory seems as if it's stored in the body rather than in the brain. Ice skaters and dancers, for example, perform without consciously thinking about which movement comes next. The body seems to just know the sequence of the routines and dances and the ability to perform the movements looks automatic—after years of practice, of course.

All automatic movement is rooted in kinesthetic memory, sometimes referred to as implicit memory. When we learned to walk, we were training the brain as well as the muscles. This task, learned in infancy, is a good example of the trial and error involved in learning movement and balance. A baby will take a few steps and then balance changes and the baby falls over. Because there is a drive to keep trying, eventually the baby walks, runs, jumps, dances, and so forth. Learning to ride a bicycle involves trial and error, too, as does driving a car. But once learned, the movements required are not forgotten. You might feel "rusty" if you have not danced the tango in a few years, but you remember the steps and eventually they again seem automatic.

If you become conscious of your movements, such as the way your arms swing when you walk, you are not necessarily improving your kinesthetic memory but you are activating your consciousness about its complexity. The next time you swim or drive, do the following:

> *Think about each move you make as you make it— the number of muscles you use in your arms and legs with each stroke across the pool and the way you automatically coordinate your head movements and your breathing. The rhythm in your movements as you glide through the water is part of kinesthetic memory. Change your stroke and notice the changes in the sensations in your body.*
>
> *After settling into the driver's seat, note every movement from putting the key in the ignition, shifting into reverse, looking in your mirrors or twisting your head to look around before you turn the wheel and accelerate. As you enter the street, become conscious of your eye movements and how often you glance at the side mirrors and rearview mirror. Are you listening? Can you hear the engine or perhaps a subtle noise when you brake? After you drive a block or two you will realize how many small actions are involved in your driving skill. This smooth, well-coordinated system is firmly entrenched in kinesthetic memory, allowing you to think about your grocery list or a client you're going to see as you drive. Unless traffic conditions demand your full attention, you can sing along to the radio, listen to language tapes, or catch up on the latest news while you safely drive.*

Spatial Memory—Where Am I? Or, Why Is This Here?

Spatial memory is related to our sense of place. Some people can glance at a map and have a good sense about where they are and how to navigate to another location. They can transfer or "translate" the information on the map to its location in the world. These individuals never get lost when they travel to a new place. The directions make perfect sense to them, and some of these people do not appear to need clear directions or maps. They just sense where they are. Some of the rest of us get lost just walking a few blocks down the street. Or, as my wife puts it, I'd get lost going to my own funeral! (You may have noticed that some people show little understanding to those who do not share their particular aptitudes.) The Japanese, as a group, have much better three-dimensional recall than the U.S. population does. As more research accumulates, other groups with this superior type of memory may be discovered.

This type of memory varies widely among individuals and perhaps among the sexes too. Based on evolutionary theory, men are better at remembering routes that cover long distances, perhaps because they were the hunters and needed to cover large areas to find food. Women appear to be superior at remembering landmarks and they can navigate without a map if they know what they should see along the way. In one of her humorous poems, Dorothy Parker wrote, "Women and elephants never forget!" It appears that elephants, like women, have a good memory for landmarks and they navigate efficiently through their territory based on familiar signs and signals along the way.

If you want to improve your spatial memory, try the following:

+ *Practice reading maps and figuring distances between destinations. Note the landmarks, towns, national parks, rivers, and so forth along the route. For short distances, memorize the streets you will cross from your home to your destination. Note bridges, stores, restaurants, bus stops, etc. Become conscious of traveling north and turning east, rather than thinking only of right and left.*

+ *With major hazards removed, close your eyes and walk from your living room to your bedroom and note how many steps you take and what you touch along the way. This exercise in "blindness" helps you sense the space around you and become familiar with your surroundings in a different way.*

+ *Draw a map of your route from home to work without looking at a real map. Note as many streets and landmarks as you can.*

Seeing in Three Dimensions

Spatial memory includes such things as understanding three-dimensional space and systems. Here too, some individuals appear to be more gifted in this area than others—I happen to be one of the less gifted. In medical school, one of the most difficult areas of anatomy for me to learn involved the three-dimensional layers of the body. For example, when we cut into a cadaver in order to learn where the arteries and nerves cross the body from front to back, it was difficult for me to absorb this information, even though I excelled in other areas of medical study.

More recently, another experience showed me a different type of spatial memory. I was on a cross-country flight, and one of the crew developed chest pains. A flight attendant asked if there was a physician on board, and I went to the cockpit to examine the woman. (As it turned out, she was having an anxiety reaction, which quickly resolved when we gave her orange juice and oxygen.)

After tending to the crewmember, I had an opportunity to chat with the pilot and look at the cockpit instrumentation. I was particularly interested in how the pilots were able to determine their exact location, based on altitude, mountain terrain, and landmarks on the ground. It struck me that it was similar to what medical students learn in pathology class. We learned to identify cells based on their patterns, rather than by how a single cell appears. Eventually, these cell patterns become part of memory. This involves spatial memory, of course, but pattern recognition is a specific kind of memory.

Pattern Memory Involves More Than Facts

Unconsciously, you see patterns when you meet people for the first time. Sometimes this has a positive overtone, but other times it can have negative results. For example, if your mother had blue eyes and red hair and a warm personality, you might recognize the pattern in other people and respond positively to redheads with the same color eyes, even before you know anything about that person. On the other hand, if you know a green-eyed brunette who is mean and narcissistic, you may see another person with similar physical characteristics and assume that person will behave the same way.

This kind of evaluation is not rational, of course, but your recognition of patterns is often unconscious and has nothing to do with logic or reason. Eventually, you may change your impression when you have facts with which to evaluate a person. Until then, your memory of patterns is dominant.

Patterns, Projection, and Homesickness

Memory patterns explain one mechanism of homesickness. I recall this phenomenon when I left home for the first time to attend college. At first, I saw people I thought I recognized from my hometown, and I would sometimes call out the name of a person, only to realize I was wrong and was seeing patterns in other people similar to the people I knew back home. My projection reflected a desire for the familiar and is an example of the way homesickness manifests. As I adjusted to college life, I no longer projected these pattern memories, my past experiences, onto reality.

In psychotherapy, we see a similar projection mechanism when patients transfer memory patterns in the form of ideas and impressions onto the therapist. A patient may form an idea, which is in essence a projection, of how the therapist thinks and behaves, based on past memory patterns. The therapist's job is to remain neutral as these projections—called transference—occur. As therapy progresses, patients come to realize that these projections are unrealistic and are based on their own memories and expectations, which in turn are based on past patterns. In this way, behavior and thought patterns eventually change.

Filling in the Blanks

Memory patterns allow us to perceive what isn't there. If I show you a long passage from a familiar work like the Gettysburg Address or John F. Kennedy's inaugural speech, but omitted a connecting word, such as "an" or "but" here and there, or I if misspelled familiar words, your pattern memory would likely insert the missing word or ignore the misspelling. Your pattern memory allows you to change the reality on the page. I recall going to Robot World in the Wisconsin Dells, which featured various activities, water parks, and so forth. One section had signs posted and the challenge was to figure out what was wrong with them. One octagonal red sign said "SLOP," which the mind fills in to read "STOP." In order to spot the mistake, we have to consciously remove the bias, so we put memory patterns aside.

Proofreaders are very familiar with the bias toward filling in what we already know to be correct. This is why some proof-readers will proof material from back to front or left to right. Changing the pattern allows them to set aside bias. Likewise, magicians can fool a crowd with their illusions because those watching bring their memory patterns to the show and project what they are used to seeing on the experience.

Nowadays we're often told that computers are in some ways "smarter" or more accurate than humans, but the truth is, humans are far better at pattern recognition than computers. Pattern recognition is one way we remember and place things in an underlying framework. When we expand the framework, we are able to expand our recognition abilities and our memory.

In general, it is easier to recognize than to identify. When patients are tested for their olfactory ability, many are able to recognize an odor. They tell us it is familiar, but they can't tell us what the odor is. This is called the "tip of the nose" syndrome, and it is similar to the "tip of the tongue" phenomenon we experience with words. If we provide patients with additional cues, such as by classifying the odor as something to eat, this helps an individual identify the odorant.

Pattern recognition is also involved in the way fears and even phobias develop. For example, if a person has an experi-ence of becoming anxious in a crowd, perhaps from a fear of being crushed, that experienced is stored as a memory. The next time the person encounters a crowd—a pattern—the fear may return, even if there is no perceived danger. However, the pattern recognition triggered the fear. The fear is not based on a rational evaluation, but memory recall is not necessarily controlled by the intellect. We tend to think it is because we associate memory with recall of facts, but emotional memory is just as significant in our lives.

Time and Sequence Memory

You have probably noticed that some people can remember birthdays and anniversaries better than others. They are able, without benefit of lists and computer reminders, to remember their father's upcoming birthday or that their wedding anniversary is a week away. These individuals *never* send one of those "belated" birthday cards or rush around at the last minute looking for a store that sells flowers and cards.

These individuals may also have an accurate internal "clock." They know what time it is without wearing a watch. They pace themselves throughout a day and generally have a sense of how much time has passed. These individuals may choose not to wear a watch for fear that they will distort their own sense of time.

Sequential memory is the ability to recall the order of things. Everyday life is filled with examples of tasks that involve sequential memory. We toast a bagel or make a bed or power up the computer by following steps in sequence, which once learned are generally automatic and require little concentration. We also recall the past based on the sequence of events, which often requires some conscious digging into our memory. Did you go to France before or after you finished sophomore year? Or was it junior year? Did you move into that house when you were 32 or 35 years old? Usually, you make other associations to help you piece together the sequence of events or steps. Sequential memories for performed tasks are generally more accurate than trying to remember the sequence of events in the past. Your life story may seem indelible but it is highly susceptible to suggestion and change.

Learn to understand your sequential memory in the following ways:

◆ *Perform a routine task out of sequence and note if it feels odd. Do you always put the water in the coffeepot before you fill the grounds basket? Switch the order and put the pot in a different place. Do this with all your routine tasks.*

◆ *Think about every trip you took away from your hometown. Make a list of vacation travels starting with the earliest and put them in order year by year. You will probably be surprised by the number of associations you must come up with in order to complete the list. In order to recall the sequence of travel events, you may need to recall where you lived, who you lived with, all your schools and jobs, your children's births, perhaps even the deaths of important people in your life—maybe even the car you drove or who won the World Series in a particular year. If this exercise is easy for you, you may have good time and sequence memory.*

Emotional Memory

Emotional memory is rooted in the instincts. For example, if someone scratches on a chalkboard with their fingernails, most people become hyper-awake, alert, and on edge—they may even perspire if the sound goes on long enough. I have this reaction when Marissa, my nine-year-old, takes two pieces of Styrofoam and rubs them together to produce a high tone. This certainly doesn't make rational sense. Most of us have never been attacked by a chalkboard. Styrofoam is not known to jump out of bushes and pounce on innocent people! Yet, we have a typical fight-or-flight response to these tones. This response to a high-pitched tone is nearly universal. The question is, Why?

The reaction to these sounds that we describe as "making our skin crawl" is not a learned response. I would suggest that the response to these tones is an instinctual memory. It could be that there was an evolutionary need for the response that is no longer needed today. But the brain doesn't know that this response is, in a sense, obsolete.

In a similar way, odors induce emotions by relying on instinctual memory in the absence of logical reasons. Odors induce an emotional response or evoke emotional memories by stimulating the right hemisphere of the brain, where emotions and odors are primarily processed. Emotional associations with odors are responsible for nostalgic reactions to smells and also may influence buying habits, the choice of a lover, or even the emotional climate at your dinner table. Based on a body of research about learning and odors, we know that certain smells can help you learn and retain information as well as recall it later. If you are using the bookmark that is offered free with this book, you may have experienced this for yourself.

You may have pleasant associations with products based on their odor as much as on their function and performance. You may link a particular lemon-scented furniture polish with the way your living room smelled when you were young. You buy the same furniture polish today, but not because it is necessarily a superior product. You have a positive emotional response to it and have developed a form of "brand loyalty."

Musical Memory

The ability to remember tones, rhythms, and chords is inherently different from the ability to remember words. When I was in medical school at the University of Michigan, I worked at a stroke rehabilitation facility evenings and weekends. We ate with the patients, many of whom had lost the ability to speak. One my fellow students, John O'Brien, worked with me; usually we had our meals with 20 or 30 patients and were the only ones who could carry on a conversation. These patients would often stay in this facility for two or three months, and over that time many gradually regained their ability to speak. The speech therapists working with these patients often used a technique called *melodic intonation therapy*, which helps retrain the brain and restore speech.

When a stroke affects the left hemisphere of the brain, where language is processed, patients often become aphasic, meaning that the ability to put appropriate words together in a logical sequence is lost and language skills must be relearned. (A stroke that affects the left hemisphere of the brain affects the right side of the body and partial paralysis also may result.)

Language skills may be relearned through music in melodic intonation therapy, because the right side of the brain processes musical memory. I observed stroke patients singing their words to communicate; they were able to sing because they activated the part of the brain unaffected by the stroke. So, these patients who were unable to have a normal conversation could sing "Happy Birthday," and eventually sing the words they wanted to speak to the tune of that simple song or others, such as "Three Blind Mice." With practice, they could sing less and use regular speech more. This therapy has great implications for learning, as well as for rehabilitation from strokes. It also demonstrates that the brain is not static; it adapts and can relearn what has been lost.

Music developed early in human culture. Written music was a much later development, so as a society's oral history depended on lexical memory, musical tradition depended on those with superior musical memory—those who were capable of passing it on to the next generation. Because singing involves both language and music, many of us hear a few notes of a melody and the words to a song immediately come back to us, even if we haven't heard or thought about the song in decades. This typically happens with the popular music of our youth. We might wonder why, if we can remember these trivial songs, we can't recall the Spanish verb forms or mathematical formulas we learned in high school.

Engaging Musical Memory

When we involve both hemispheres of the brain and more than one sensory system, we have a better chance to retain information. For this reason, if we hear, read, and write a fact, we are more likely to remember it. If we add music, the emotional brain is engaged as well, and this enhances learning. I once heard about a teacher who assigned a list of spelling words that his students had to learn every week. Not only were the students instructed to learn to spell the words, they had to reconstruct the list of twenty words from memory. This was an unusual way to teach spelling, and most of the students found it very difficult. However, one student put the list of words to music (she chose a familiar spiritual with a strong beat), and when it came time to take the test, she remembered every word. Other students, and the teacher, too, wondered how she managed to do so well on these spelling tests. When she told the others about her "trick," most thought it sounded so ridiculous they wouldn't try it. But without fully understanding the reason behind it, this student created a memory device that engaged musical memory and, hence, both hemispheres of the brain. The lesson we can learn here is that *if it's important to move a certain set of facts into memory storage, match the facts with music.*

We are all familiar with some forms of musical memory. If you need to remember if "m" comes before "n" or if "w" comes after "v," you might need to sing the alphabet song all the way through, but the information is there. It never fails! You know that September, April, June, and November are 30 days long because the song you hum in your head serves as a reminder you can call up whenever you need it.

Most of us can improve memory and learning with music, but a few individuals are unable to learn information from music because they have no musical memory, a condition called *amusia.* These individuals can process spoken language and other sounds, but the pleasure of music eludes them.

The Familiar Numbers

Numerical memory is an additional type of memory, and like language, numbers are symbols. We usually remember numbers in sequence for a particular purpose—phone numbers, addresses, birthdays, and so forth. Most people process numerical memory in the dominant, or left, hemisphere. Some people have an aptitude for mathematics and numerical memory. I once memorized the formula for the mathematical symbol for pi to its twenty-fifth decimal place. I did this when I was locked out of my house one afternoon and I had to sit on the front stairs and wait for my mother to come home. I had my math book with me, and although there was no practical value to memorizing this piece of mathematical information, it was a way for me to pass the time.

Other young people might have chosen to pass the time in a physically active way or by reciting poems or singing songs in their head. Some children may have simply engaged in some fanciful daydreaming. But I have an aptitude for numerical memory and I chose this way to occupy myself while I waited. Our aptitudes influence personality characteristics and our choices, even those as trivial as how we might spend a few idle minutes.

Learning: Seeing, Hearing, Feeling

At one time, the variations in what has come to be called "learning style" were given scanty attention. Perceptive teachers understood that their students learned in different ways, but generally, educational systems were designed around reading, which is advantageous for visual learners, but not necessarily for students with other dominant learning styles. Three dominant learning styles discussed here are visual learning, learning by hearing, and learning by doing (kinesthetic learning).

Visual images are processed very quickly, and in many people the link between visual learning and memory is strong. Most of us are better at recognizing faces than we are at remembering names, for example. However, if we read a name and see a face, we have a better chance of connecting the name to the face.

The term *prosopagnosia* refers to a condition in which a person has no memory for faces at all. Prosopagnosics are obviously socially handicapped and must find ways to compensate for this disability. As a guest on the Jerry Springer show, I met a woman who must tell the people she meets that she will not recognize them if she sees them again and assure them that her lack of response is not meant to be insulting. Her friends and family have learned to adjust and she lives quite normally, but prosopagnosia is undoubtedly a handicap in business and social settings.

Visual learners tend to express themselves in language that

reflect their predominate style. They might say, "Oh, I see your point," or, "My view is different from yours." Visual memory also involves geographic memory. Those with good geographic memory are able to determine direction. Stand on any street and ask them to point to north or south, and chances are they will be right.

Eidetic memory is photographic memory, meaning that the person retains visual information in precise form. Those few individuals with photographic memory are able to recreate words on a page after one reading. It has been suggested that about 50 percent of children have eidetic memory up to age ten or so, after which this ability begins to fade. Some adults, however, appear to retain a superior visual memory and can recite previously read information fairly accurately.

Some individuals learn quickly by hearing information. These individuals would rather hear a story than read a novel; in general, they retain information by listening to it. They can listen to directions and generally don't need a map in order to find their way. Verbal instructions are sufficient. They tend to tell you that they "hear" what you're saying, or their facial expressions may reflect careful listening.

Kinesthetic learning represents a third category of learning. These individuals often show a preference for learning by doing. In high school biology class, the kinesthetic learners were eager to dissect the frog and as children they liked to take things apart to see how they work. This type of learning goes beyond physical activity, however. Kinesthetic learners tend to be intuitive and receive their cues from the body. For example, they may pick up on body language more quickly than others, and these individuals use expressions such as, "This just feels right," or, "I sense that you and I don't agree." When former President Clinton used the phrase, "I feel your pain," he was using a kinesthetic expression. He didn't say, "I hear your distress," or "I can see you're having trouble." The phrase he chose reflects his personal communication style.

Although we need to recognize that some people have clear predominance of one type of learning style, we all share these styles to a degree. Physical activities, from walking to hitting a home run or dunking a basketball, involve kinesthetic memory. Learning to read involves visual learning and memory, and spoken language and music are dependent on auditory learning and memory. Given the range of skills most of us use every day, it is clear that we use multiple kinds of learning and memory styles to function. And most of the time we do not give these styles much thought.

One day, we may be able to accurately correlate dominant learning styles with other personality characteristics. For example, a child who spends idle minutes doing math calculations may have a specific learning style that correlates with other personality traits. In my last book, *What Flavor is Your Personality?*, I reported findings from numerous studies that linked food preferences, in other words, snack foods, spices, ice cream flavors, and so forth, with personality types. Based on the results of this research, I believe that one day we will be able to predict what kind of learning style is dominant in your personality based on your preference for one snack food over another. Or, we may be able to correlate your food preferences with your dominant abilities, such as numerical versus an artistic bent.

Eventually, we may find links between such things as color preferences, odor and food preferences, learning styles, intellectual aptitudes, leadership and management styles, and so forth. Thus far, research in these areas has been promising. We can safely say that our personality leaves an imprint on everything we do, even the way we tie our shoes or learn a language or drive a car.

Do You Remember Where You Were When...?

The Far Side creator, Gary Larson, captured the nature of a special kind of memory in one of his cartoons. The picture showed a group of animals gathered together in the forest talking about where they were when they heard the news that Bambi's mother had been shot. Anyone who has ever seen Disney's *Bambi* will immediately relate.

Every generation has experienced events that are so far out of the ordinary that the memory of them does not appear to fade with time. Each individual has a unique "picture" of what was happening at the moment the news of the event was heard, hence the term "flashbulb" memory. Just think how many millions of people in our country can tell you exactly where they were when they heard that President John Kennedy was shot or the World Trade Center had been attacked.

I was in second grade when President Kennedy was shot, yet I can vividly recall that I was watching *Bozo's Circus* on television while I was eating my lunch. My older brother, Steven, told me that the president had been shot and I knew from his tone of voice that something of great significance had happened. I remember that I was eating a hamburger and the kitchen table was white, and all the other visual details of the scene are clear, as if, as the saying goes, the event happened yesterday. Actually, this event is far more clear to me than many of yesterday's insignificant events. Millions of men and women have a flashbulb memory of that and other events that are remembered as crises.

Many individuals in my parents' generation recall precisely where they were and what was happening the moment they heard about the bombing of Pearl Harbor in 1941. Some people have a flashbulb memory of Martin Luther King's assassination or of the Challenger space shuttle explosion. More recently, many of us have a flashbulb memory of the Oklahoma City bombing and the September 11 tragedy.

The flashbulb phenomenon was noted and documented by an early psychologist, F.W. Colgrove, who, in 1899, interviewed individuals who were alive when President Lincoln was shot. Each individual had a unique memory of where they were and what they were doing, and for each individual the memories were detailed and vivid, with the surrounding sensory details intact, even after thirty-four years.

The phenomenon of flashbulb memory tends to be associated with a collective crisis. There is a strong element of shock involved, of course, because no one is prepared for assassinations, bombings, and or disasters of enormous proportions or import. By definition, we cannot anticipate these moments. Psychologist Roger Livingstone suggests that we are neurologically "wired" to imprint such events. It's as if a signal is released in the brain that says, "Now Print."

As accurate as flashbulb memories seem to be, they can be distorted by time just as other memories change. The "Now Print" mechanism isn't perfect. The accuracy of flashbulb memories has been tested by asking participants to record their memories shortly after the event and again weeks or months later. The details do change after all. In other words, your memory of one of our pivotal national crises may not be quite as accurate as you think it is. The table in the kitchen of my childhood home might not have been white after all.

Absolute accuracy aside, the phenomenon of the flashbulb memory takes on increasing significance as constantly improved communications make the world "smaller." A patient of mine told me that he is startled every time he hears the music and sees the image on television that indicates "breaking news." For him, the fear that another leader has been assassinated immediately surfaces and the memories of past tragedies are recalled. His experience is probably quite common nowadays, which shows how certain words and images induce a conditioned response. The kind of events that take on global significance has also been redefined. Who would have predicted that the death of Princess Diana would have been an event that produced hundreds of millions of flashbulb memories?

Try this exercise and keep what you record in order to test it later for accuracy:

> *Make a list of your flashbulb memories and write down all the detail you recall: place, time, smells, colors, sounds, the other people with you, what was happening in your life, and so forth. Write quickly—do not consider the details too carefully. You may be surprised by how many flashbulb memories you have. You may also note that yours are not the same as those of others around you. For example, you may have a flashbulb memory of the moment the Gulf War began, but the death of Princess Diana is not a prominent flashbulb memory. Later, ask friends and family what they recall about these "Now Print" moments. You may find many similarities and differences.*

Thirty Seconds, Thirty Minutes, Thirty Years

In neurology, we have traditionally divided memory into *immediate*, *recent*, and *remote*. In popular literature, these classifications are sometimes referred to as *short-term* or *long-term* memory.

Immediate memory is the ability to recall information just after receiving it. For example, patients being tested for immediate recall ability will be asked to repeat digits forward and backward. We usually start with seven random numbers—9381047, for example. If a patient can recall seven numbers, we discontinue the test. If not, we try six numbers, then five, and so forth.

Most adults are able to retain the memory of seven numbers for a few seconds. If the number is of no importance, it is then forgotten and is not transferred to long-term storage. You can call information—411—from a pay phone and if you repeat the number the operator recites, you can usually remember it long enough to dial it. The sound of an ambulance siren, for example, can be distracting enough that the seven digits are either lost or confused—is it 9381047 or 9381074? Try adding a tune to the numbers as you repeat them and see if you have an easier time remembering them. (The first bar of "Happy Birthday" adapts well to the seven-digit phone number.)

Seven appears to a kind of magic number. Most adults can consistently retain seven items or numbers and repeat them back. Relatively few adults can consistently retain more, and a few individuals are unable to go beyond five or six. It is no accident that phone numbers, not counting the area code, are seven digits. It is a number that suits a common capability for immediate recall. This capacity differs among cultures, however. While seven digits are compatible for short-term memory capabilities in the U.S., in China the population can generally retain more numbers.

We have a different system for transferring sequential numbers and items into permanent storage. If we really want to remember a series of numbers, such as our Social Security number, we break it up into sections. We also break words into syllables when we spell them, particularly aloud. This is called *chunking*. Our Social Security number is divided into three parts: 3 digits, 2 digits, and 4 digits. It has a certain rhythm when we repeat it. Our phone number has two parts, and a third if we add the area code. We think of the number in chunks—and usually recite it in chunks as well.

Recent recall is the ability to recall information received in the very recent past. For example, when testing patients for recent recall ability, we will name four objects and the patient will repeat them back to us. Then the patient is distracted for about three minutes, then is asked to repeat the names of the objects. If the person is unable to remember the items, then a cue is given. If one of the items is "tulip," the cue might be, "The item is a flower." Memory is much improved by offering a cue, which suggests that this is a powerful tool to enhance recall of any stored information. Impairment in recent recall is associated with the presence of certain disorders, such as Wernicke-Korsakoff syndrome, a condition common in alcoholics.

Remote memory is what is commonly spoken of as long-term memory. Remote memory includes everything we know and it is why we can distinguish a tulip from a rose and the fragrance of cinnamon rolls from the stench of a toxic waste dump. From infancy, you were developing the information that is now part of your remote memory. When an infant crawls across the floor picking at the carpet or reaching for a toy, he or she is developing motor skills and is learning by seeing and touching. Babies put everything in their mouths in order to learn the range of tastes and smells in their environment. All the skills you perform automatically are imprinted in the brain in long-term storage. Emotions are imprinted, too, of course, as are our complex impressions of the world and the connections we make between concepts and information.

Classifications and Associations

The ability to classify and categorize information is one of brain's most important skills. Once we know the category "flower," we can think of all the flowers we know, and we know that carrots and potatoes are not flowers, but belong to another category of information. We can further subcategorize, as young children may observe and then classify the information that daffodils are spring flowers and marigolds stay in bloom into the fall. One of the earliest tests in school, even preschool, measures a child's ability to recognize the familiar things in the world that "go together." Rabbit, chipmunk, and raccoon go together, but seagull doesn't fit.

The ability to make associations allows abstract thinking. For example, we can take abstract concepts such as freedom or patriotism, and through association we might begin to think about the Declaration of Independence, the Bill of Rights, the flag, the Civil War, Abraham Lincoln, Martin Luther King, and so on. Or, any one of these concrete ideas may start associations with abstract concepts.

Basic Ways of Learning

We often think that learned information is valuable because it allows us to analyze complex information and create new things, from novels and poems and dance steps to computer programs and mathematical formulas and surgical procedures. This is certainly true, but much of what we need to know to get along in the world is conditioned learning.

Classical conditioning was studied by the Russian physiologist, Ivan Pavlov, whose famous dogs learned to salivate at the sound of a bell. Pavlov noted that dogs begin to salivate at the sight of food or when they smell it. To the dogs, these stimuli signaled that a meal would soon follow and their salivary glands responded. Pavlov then became curious if a neutral signal, followed by food, could also trigger salivation. Eventually, as you probably know, Pavlov's dogs were conditioned to salivate at the sound of a bell if dinner soon followed. Hence, the dogs showed a conditioned response and the bell was the conditioning stimulus.

Pavlov, who had originally set out to research digestion, eventually won a Nobel Prize for explaining the components of a conditioned response. His experiments have been repeated many times with a variety of laboratory animals. There are many variations on the theme of conditioned response, but in general, we can say that much of our behavior, including salivating when the odor of food is presented, are based on prior conditioning. If you begin to feel hungry when you inhale the odor of apple pie, you are responding to conditioning. The centers in the brain that control hunger and satiety are conditioned to respond to certain food odors. Food aversions operate in a similar way. I once became ill after eating curried chicken, and although this experience occurred many years ago, I still am unable to eat curried dishes of any kind. This isn't rational, but I have been conditioned to associate curry with illness, and my conditioning happened with only one negative experience.

Our response to the sound of a ringing telephone is another kind of conditioned response. We do not need to relearn that the bell signals the telephone. The buzzer on the microwave and the shrill sound of your alarm clock also stimulate a conditioned or habitual response.

Conditioned responses can be helpful and save us mental energy and time, but they can also be negative. For example, Jim, a patient of mine, had difficulty getting along with his boss, who was a critical and domineering presence in the office. Eventually, the sound of the boss' footsteps coming down the hall caused Jim to feel tense, including the physical responses to stress. His heart rate increased and he had an uneasy sensation in his solar plexus. Even thinking about his boss could cause this conditioned response. Deconditioning could take place only if the boss changed his ways or if Jim consciously changed his attitude toward the boss and his job—or if he found another job. It was interesting that once Jim decided to leave that company and began to search for a new job, his response to the boss changed, even before he gave his notice and left. The perception that an encounter would be negative was removed when Jim no longer cared about his boss' reactions to him.

The point is that learned responses can be changed when we choose to. For example, some treatments for phobias involve changing the conditioned response to the stimulus that triggers the fear. This is deconditioning or desensitizing therapy. (The development of an extreme fear is itself a conditioned response.)

State-dependent learning, discussed in chapter 1, represents a form of conditioning. For example, if you study for a math test while you eat chocolate, you will recall more if you eat chocolate during the actual test. Odors associated with learning have been shown to have an effect on recall. State-dependent learning can even operate in inebriated states. Studies have shown that information learned after consuming alcohol—even in amounts large enough to make the study subjects drunk—is later recalled more easily when the subjects again consumed alcohol. The scented bookmark, however, is a much safer way to introduce state-dependent learning, so forget the alcohol and bring out the bookmark!

Operant conditioning involves the many systems of consequences in the form of rewards, punishments, and reinforcement with which we are all familiar. When you consistently remove your children from the living room if they misbehave, you are conditioning them to stick to the rules you have established. (At least you hope this will happen.) Breaking a habit such as cigarette smoking is likely to be more effective if you set up a system of rewards that help to reinforce your commitment. Some smoking cessation programs suggest taking the money that one would have spent on cigarettes in a week or a month and using it for something special or prized, such as clothing or a massage or a special book or tape. Weight loss programs often offer similar advice.

All the systems we have that offer prizes, trophies, certificates, and so forth are basically created to provide positive conditioning. Praising children when they do something correctly is nothing more than a form of operant conditioning. A schedule of raises and promotions in the workplace is another form of operant conditioning, which reinforces desired behavior. Much of human behavior can be traced to ongoing systems of operant conditioning.

Operant conditioning has other implications. For example, many psychologists believe that beyond the superficial systems of rewards and punishments and reinforcements we are familiar with, operant conditioning influences the kind of society we create. Children who grow up in severely dysfunctional homes or communities may learn that nothing they do produces positive consequences and there is no escape from negative events. Learned helplessness is a term used to describe a situation in which an individual has no sense of control over the environment. Children born into what has been called the underclass in our country are at risk of feeling and behaving in a helpless and resigned manner. At an early age, they may believe they have no control over their circumstances, and as a result of this learned helplessness they are conditioned to accept a life of poverty and lack of opportunity. (Remember the shock among our population when some children growing up in communities in which considerable violence had taken place began using the phrase "If I grow up," rather than "When I grow up.") Contrast this situation with the operant conditioning of children in more privileged environments who are repeatedly told that if they do certain things, their future is in their own hands.

Observational learning is our ability to learn from watching others and internalizing expected consequences. Most of us were not formally taught to wash dishes or get ready for work in the morning. We learned these skills or expected routines from watching other people. Our "odor" behavior is learned largely through observation. For example, some children learn that perfumes and aftershave lotions are reserved for special occasions; others learn that such fragrances are used every day. Some children learn to inhale the odor of food and comment on the fragrance before eating; in other families, such behavior would be considered rude. To many individuals, telling another person that he or she smells good may be normal social behavior, but to others, it may be far too intimate a comment for most social interactions.

Throughout childhood we also learn from the consequences that we (or others) experience as a result of their behavior. Most of us figure out fairly early that stealing is not acceptable. We may learn this because an older sibling stole something and the consequences were very negative. We may learn that lying is unacceptable most of the time, but is okay in other situations. It is acceptable to tell your hosts that you love their furniture even if you don't, because social interactions require less than frank truth.

This kind of learning is dependent on societal expectations and is subject to change. When I was a child, it was considered impolite to ask an injured or disabled person about their crutches or wheelchair. Most parents reinforced the notion that such questions would make the injured or disabled person uncomfortable and might even cause hurt feelings. In many situations, it was not even considered acceptable to offer help. One result was that disabled individuals often felt isolated and the whole subject became taboo in public or social situations. Today, there is a more enlightened atmosphere, and children are less likely to have their natural curiosity discouraged and the issues of illness and disability are discussed more openly. This is just one example where attitudes have changed and observational learning reinforces shifting attitudes.

The above descriptions are by necessity brief and, in actuality, all forms of learning are complex and not entirely predictable. Human behavior cannot be neatly controlled. However, these concepts will be expanded upon in various chapters of this book and many are directly or indirectly influenced by odors in the environment.

Do Not Bore Your Brain

You may love your routines, but your brain likes novelty. The brain likes the opportunity to learn new information or perform familiar tasks in a different way. As you have seen thus far, we learn, store, and organize information in a variety of ways, and the more we engage our senses in our observation and learning processes, the more we retain. As we mature and settle into patterns and routines—we could call them "ruts"—we may need to consciously remind ourselves to shake things up a little. Remind yourself to learn in new ways and engage the "novelty factor" in your daily activities.

Sharpen Your Ability to Memorize

Remember the feeling you had when you knew a poem or an important list or a Bible passage "by heart." Except for some childhood songs and nursery rhymes (which often seem almost *too* easily recalled), most of us know very few poems or famous speeches or documents by heart. Memorization may or may not have a tangible value, but the exercise itself is a form of mental aerobics. Besides, you'll impress your friends when you casually drop lines of poetry or philosophical gems into the conversation!

So, pick a favorite poem or an important document, such as the Declaration of Independence or the Bill of Rights, and get started.

1. Choose a place in your home or office where you will practice memorizing, preferably every day, but two or three times a week is also valuable.

2. Choose an odor that you will associate with the place and the task. Use that ambient odor in the air each time you begin. You could use air freshener, a scented candle, or aromatic oil in a diffuser. Just be sure to use the same odor in the same place in your office or home every day.

3. Divide the piece you are memorizing into chunks, in other words, learn one four-line verse of a poem or one amendment in the Bill of Rights or a few Bible verses each session. You are now practicing, and this stage of learning is known as the "rehearsal" stage.

4. At the beginning of each session, practice reciting what you memorized before.

5. Use as many sensory associations as you can to help you remember. Recite the piece outloud. Form pictures of the material in your head. Stand up and use gestures, as the great orators have always done. These gestures add kinesthetic cues. Elocution was once taught in schools, and recitation was considered a performance art, so get your hands and body moving when you practice.

6. Strive to overlearn. The reason you know the Pledge of Allegiance, the National Anthem, and "Humpty-Dumpty" is that you have heard these words — and their rhythms — so many times that you can't forget. Repetition is key to memorization.

7. Encourage your children to memorize — make it a family game. They may balk and tell you it's too hard or boring — or worse. Ignore their protests and encourage it anyway. It's good for their brain development.

The Novelty Factor I—A Game of Firsts

Most of us remember "firsts." We can recall details about our first job, first love, first trip to Europe, and first car. Runners remember their first marathon, but have to think about their fourth or fifth. The novelty factor is what makes "firsts" so memorable.

Develop your personal book of firsts. What are your associations with these memories? Recall the sensory details, including the smells. How did these experiences shape your life? You'll learn a lot about yourself and what has had meaning in your life when you think about your personal firsts. Develop a personal autobiography by recalling these first-time experiences.

Here are some samples to get you started:

What Do I Recall About My First:

- ✦ day of school
- ✦ book I read by myself
- ✦ childhood friend
- ✦ vacation or trip with my parents
- ✦ trip abroad
- ✦ bedroom
- ✦ move from one home to another

- ✦ athletic event
- ✦ hobby or special interest
- ✦ movie I saw
- ✦ date
- ✦ love
- ✦ important loss
- ✦ date with my current partner
- ✦ job
- ✦ kiss
- ✦ sex
- ✦ day of college
- ✦ day of my honeymoon
- ✦ day on each job I've had
- ✦ time I was fired
- ✦ speech or presentation
- ✦ major goal reached

As you can see, your life is filled with firsts, but at the same time, many of the experiences that you considered unforgettable have receded deep into your memory. For example, you may have had a fabulous time on your honeymoon or on your first trip to Japan or France, but can you remember the third day or the fifth day? Chances are that you recall the first day more vividly than all others. Similarly, if you've ever been fired from a job, you may remember your first day on the job and the day you were fired, but the other days just run together.

The Novelty Factor II — Break Out of Your Rut

Keep your brain sharp by consciously introducing change into your life. You may believe change is difficult and try to avoid it, but your brain "perks up" when you alter even minor patterns in your life. Engage all your senses as you:

+ Take a different route to work.

+ Sit in a different section of the commuter train or bus.

+ Try a new food.

+ Dress up your dining room table with flowers or eat in a different room.

+ Shop at a new store to break the routine.

+ Listen to a new type of music.

+ Introduce a new scent into your home.

+ Wear a new scent.

+ Use your nondominant hand to perform a simple task, such as making coffee or buttoning your shirt or blouse.

+ Wear a color you have never worn before.

+ If you work in a field that engages your left brain, try activities that use your right brain—leave the performance reports at work and listen to music or dance at home.

+ If you work in a creative field, practice a left brain activity at home. For example, balance your checkbook or learn a personal-finance accounting computer program at home. Use your bookmark to help you learn your new skill.

+ Practice a foreign language and create a state-dependent learning situation by introducing an odor to your study sessions—and put phrases and lists of verb conjugations to music and sing the words.

4

Memory, Mood, and Odors

"He saw that there was no mood of the mind that had not its counterpart in the sensuous life, and set himself to discover their true relations, wondering what there was in frankincense that made one mystical, and in ambergris that stirred one's passions, and in violets that woke the memory of dead romances, and in musk that troubled the brain. . . ."

– Oscar Wilde, *The Picture of Dorian Gray*

If concentration and motivation are critical to learning and to the ability to retain and recall information, one's mood is equally important. One's mood can determine if focused attention is possible because mood plays a role in motivation and the ability to learn. This is where our sense of smell has one of its most important roles, because it affects memory and emotions more than other senses do. Mood states have implications for the classroom, the workplace, and any environment in which it is necessary to learn new information or concentrate on a task, including, of course, social occasions. Because the sense of smell, more than any other sense, is the "emotional" sense, odors have both a direct and indirect influence on mood.

Stress, Tension, and Anxiety

Dr. J.R. King, a British psychiatrist, tells a story about passing an organic chemistry lab and enjoying the odors because he had spent so many happy hours in the lab as a young student.

Some years later he passed the lab on the way to the room where he faced stressful medical examinations, and the nostalgia evoked by the odor had a beneficial effect on his mood. King refers to his response as the "Marcel Proust phenomenon" because of the many references that Proust made in his writing to the odors that caused shifts in mood.

In studies conducted at our foundation, we have found that certain odors reduce anxiety, which is important because anxiety tends to be self-reinforcing. If you experience mild anxiety, your awareness of your anxious state tends to make you more anxious. A public speaker, for example, may become afraid that others can observe the outward signs of his or her mood state (trembling hands, shaky voice, and so forth) and that fear will make the speaker even more concerned. Anxiety in learning environments is so common that test anxiety is considered a common malady among students and, in some cases, even a "condition" in a clinical sense. Using odors in classrooms, offices, public speaking situations, or even cocktail parties has the potential to reduce anxiety, thereby preventing the anxious state from escalating.

Information about odors that may reduce anxiety and stress or lift mood comes from many sources including those who study the science of perfumery, folklore, and medical texts dating back many centuries. In sixteenth-century China, for example, the odor of rose oil was said to have antidepressant properties, and chamomile oil was used as a sedative, essentially as a way to relieve anxiety. Many people still drink chamomile tea to relax before sleep, and your grandparents may swear by its calming effects on both adults and children. Four centuries ago, European medical thinking included the belief that peppermint strengthens the brain and preserves memory. Modern scientific research has shown that the odor of jasmine stimulates beta waves in the front of the brain and tends to make one feel awake and alert, a state that promotes learning.

It is important to understand that the response to certain odors is not purely subjective, but rather that some odors act on the central nervous system in ways we can measure. In the 1970s, Paola Rovesti, a professor at the Milan University in Italy, investigated essential oils and came up with a list of potentially anxiety-reducing fragrances, including lime, marjoram, violet leaf, rose, lavender, bergamot, and cypress. Lemon, orange, verbena, jasmine, ylang-ylang, and sandalwood were shown to act against depressed mood. Others have mentioned clary sage and grapefruit for their antidepressive qualities. In some cases, the scents are described as inducing mild euphoria, rather than simply working to reverse depression.

Although I cannot recommend using *any* of these oils to treat clinical depression or chronic anxiety because consistent and effective treatments using odors are still in the future, research has documented physiologic changes in response to odors. Changes in brain wave patterns, heart rate, blood pressure, muscle tension, and skin temperature are among the documented physiological responses.

Dr. King, who has used odors in his practice, reports that his patients' initial responses to the aromas is positive. They report an overall lift in mood — feeling better, brighter, or relaxed. As Dr. King pointed out, this shift in mood did not mean that the patients' physical or psychological complaints were cured, but rather that simply "feeling better" can facilitate the healing process.

Mood and the Aroma of Food

In the 1980s research showed that the odor of nutmeg oil may help reduce stress, as evidenced by reduced systolic blood pressure readings. Study participants also reported feeling less tension, anxiety, anger, and embarrassment, as well as feeling more calm, relaxed, and happy. Additional research demonstrated that a nutmeg-apple odor increased theta wave activity (associated with relaxation) in the brain, to a greater degree than lavender or eucalyptus. Since all three odors were rated as pleasant, the difference in results may be attributable to the direct effect on the brain, or it may be that apple-nutmeg is a food odor, and as such, has a stress-reducing effect.

Food odors are known to have a powerful influence on mood. Simply imagining a favorite dessert resulted in EEG changes in study subjects that were similar to those that resulted when participants were given instructions that induce relaxation. In the male arousal study conducted by our foundation, the odor of cinnamon rolls and pumpkin pie increased penile blood flow more than the odor of any cologne. The most powerful odor for male sexual arousal was a combination of pumpkin pie and lavender. The food odors of Good and Plenty candy and cucumber also increased female sexual arousal, although no odor we introduced increased female arousal to the same degree as the male response.

The reasons for our results remain unclear. It is possible that the odors had a direct effect on the arousal center of the brain, or the smells were pleasant and may have evoked a positive mood, thereby facilitating arousal. It is also possible that response to food odors is related to our evolutionary past and makes sense in that context. Our earliest ancestors probably lived in relatively solitary groups, but gathered around food kills where food odors prevailed. During these times of "feast," the sexes likely found their chances of finding a mate increased, particularly if food odors promoted arousal for both men and women. If survival of the species is the goal, it makes sense for both sexes to be aroused by food odors and in contexts where men and women would gather together. In modern life, we tend to forget that nature is less concerned about love and romance and that the basic sexual drive is present to ensure procreation so our species survives. These aromas are in essence reaching into our evolutionary past and taking advantage of influences on sexual arousal that we may have forgotten about in our quest to appeal to the opposite sex.

Odors and Perceptions of Space

In our study of odors and claustrophobia, the odor of green apple influenced perception of room size. Our results suggested that those suffering from mild claustrophobia might be helped if the odor of green apple is introduced. The odor affects perception and the room is perceived as larger and therefore more comfortable. Based on these results, a person who experiences claustrophobia in an elevator may be helped by sniffing the odor of green apple while in the elevator.

The Smell & Taste Treatment and Research Foundation also tested the odor of green apple to determine if it had an effect on the severity of symptoms associated with migraine headaches. We assessed 60 patients during three separate migraine episodes. During one of these testing sessions, we asked participants to smell of odor of green apple, and the other two sessions served as non-odor control periods. We found reduction in severity of symptoms among individuals who had normal ability to smell and who also liked the odor. The exact mechanism is not yet clear, and we are not certain if the positive response to the odor of green apple was psychological or physiological. However, certain neurotransmitters, including serotonin, dopamine, nor-epinephrine, and beta-endorphin, are known as modulators of headaches, but are also found in the olfactory bulb. We may find many mechanisms at work, including the ability of the green apple odor to reduce blood pressure and anxiety.

The odor of heliotropin, which is a vanilla-like smell, reduced anxiety among individuals during a medical test, magnetic resonance imaging (MRI). MRI is a painless test, but it can cause anxiety because it is noisy and confining. A claustrophobic response is not uncommon. Those exposed to the heliotropin at the time of testing reported 63 percent less anxiety than those in a non-odorized environment during the test. It is possible that the odor of green apple would produce the same effect. In fact, MRI centers through the U.S. are now infusing the green apple aroma throughout their facilities.

Heading to the Beach

It is probably is no accident that the beach, particularly an ocean beach, is a favored vacation spot. For many people, a trip to the ocean can induce a profound sense of relaxation, and cares and worries seem to fall away. Apparently, physical changes mirror the psychological response, since sea odors have been found to reduce muscle contractions in the face by 20 percent. You may have noticed that sea-scented colognes, shower gels, lotions, and soaps, as well as room deodorizing sprays, are turning up on cosmetic counters. Some cosmetic companies have entire lines of these products, all marketed on the premise that the odor of the sea is by its nature relaxing. If we can't get away to the beach for a vacation, we can bring the beach home and relax in our bathroom "spa." And there is no harm in experimenting with these odors and monitoring how they make you feel.

Test and Performance Anxiety

Mild excitement or apprehension prior to a test or a performance is both common and normal. In our society, testing is a traditional part of our educational system that very few of us escape. Admission into colleges and graduate programs require testing as well. Even when school days are over, many companies perform batteries of tests on every job applicant. (The value of this extensive testing is continually debated, but so far, testing remains firmly entrenched and most people must adjust rather than try to "fight the system.")

An aroused mood state before and during a test or performance may actually have a positive influence. A bit of anxiety may put us at the "top of our game," so to speak. However, extreme test and performance anxiety is debilitating and can interfere with a student's ability to reach educational goals or an adult's ability to fulfill professional ambitions.

Since we know that certain odors reduce anxiety, it makes sense to try them as a safe remedy for test and performance anxiety. Start with food odors, such as green apple, spiced apple, nutmeg, or vanilla. Research has shown that lavender, sometimes called the "student's herb," not only promotes relaxation, but may actually help students perform mathematical calculations. If, however, lavender makes you too relaxed, then try an odor that is more stimulating such as lemon, which has been shown to help clerical workers make fewer errors, or peppermint or jasmine, both of which influence beta waves activity in the brain, thereby promoting an awake and alert state. These odors are also considered refreshing and pleasant, but they do not increase tension or anxiety. Pine is a non-food odor that has a similar effect and is used at Heathrow Airport in London to evoke a relaxed mood among passengers. For some people, pine is an especially pleasant odor and it may be relaxing enough to work as a stress reducer at exam time, perhaps because it evokes a nostalgic response.

Another strategy is to create a state-dependent learning

environment that extends to the exams. For example, if you eat chocolate mints when you have a relaxing massage, you could sniff or eat chocolate mints when you take a test. The conditioned response to the odor may be sufficient to reduce anxiety in both settings. As you can see, this is a variation on state-dependent learning and uses scents to influence a mood shift, regardless of the setting.

Since everyone is different, I cannot recommend one single odor that will work for everyone. Set up your own informal research project and test odors on yourself in settings where you want to increase relaxation and in settings and in testing and performance environments where you want to be alert and focused, but not too anxious to perform well. Use the scientific research results presented here as guidelines for your own experiments.

Lavender, Peppermint, and Concentration and Efficiency

In general, lavender is linked with relaxation and peppermint is linked with an awake and alert state. Both mental states are necessary for focused concentration. Researchers tested both odors with sixty-seven (58 women, 9 men) volunteers, who were recruited to proofread pages of text that contained misspelled words. They performed the proofreading task in three sections, once in the presence of lavender, once with peppermint diffused in the environment, and once with no odor present. (The diffuser used, by the way, was similar to those you can buy for use in your home.) Each proofreading session was thirty minutes. While the men's sample was small, they generally performed better with the odor of peppermint in the room. Overwhelmingly, the women worked more efficiently and found a greater number of spelling errors when lavender was diffused through the room than in the presence of peppermint.

This research suggests that the same odors may influence men and women differently, or that perhaps the mood state of the sexes going into the proofreading settings were different. It is possible that the men required a more alert state to perform the proofreading tasks efficiently and the women required a greater degree of relaxation to perform. When you are experimenting in your home, keep in mind that even mild anxiety about a task may influence your degree of concentration. Likewise, an alert state is required to maintain motivation and concentration. These effects may be subtle, but as you notice your shift in mood, be aware of the odors in your environment.

Lavender represents an interesting case because it enjoys wide acceptance as a relaxing odor and we found it may help elderly individuals fall asleep more easily and quickly. However, when tested, it does not appear to influence anxiety. Our foundation tested the ability of lavender to reduce anxiety during a timed arithmetic test. We had thirty subjects (college students) perform the arithmetic test in the presence of lavender odor and again in an odor-free environment. We tested our group for physiological indicators of anxiety, with three self-report measures of mood, and with a written test called the Zung Anxiety Scale. We found no measurable difference in our subjects' self-reported mood state in the presence of lavender odor, nor did the physiological measures show any change in anxiety indicators. In addition, although lavender is commonly suggested in popular aromatherapy books for use in massage oils and in other settings designed to be soothing and therapeutic, only 8 percent of our subjects reported finding the odor pleasant.

Our study did not definitively show that lavender has no value in reducing anxiety, because our subjects had not been diagnosed with generalized anxiety disorder. However, we can say that lavender is not universally appealing, nor is necessarily a positive concentration odor. For this reason, I recommend experimenting with odors rather than relying on recommendations that appear in the popular press based on assumptions that may be based on tradition and folklore but not necessarily scientific evidence. (See "Natural or Artificial Odors?" on page 106.)

Thoughts and Emotions Influence Each Other

Thoughts and emotions tend to mirror one another. If you are feeling down, you're likely to be pessimistic and see the glass as half-empty. But when your mood lifts, you are more likely to be optimistic, and now the glass is half-full. When you're happy, you are likely to think positive thoughts and happier memories.

In addition, when one's mood is positive, a wider range of information is recalled. In controlled research conditions, investigators used odors to create pleasant and unpleasant memories among a group of female college students. Later, the students were able to recall more memories in the presence of the pleasant odor of almond than in the unpleasant odor of pyridine (a chemical derived from coal tar).

Another operative principle is that it is easier to remember information that is consistent with one's current mood. So, if you are already sad, unpleasant childhood memories, for example, are more likely to surface. When you are happy, you will remember happy childhood memories. Odors that are pleasant generally lift mood, which then results in recall of more pleasant memories.

So, how happy should you be? Well, a very upbeat mood can actually interfere with the ability to process new information. This information has relevance in the sales field, for example. If a buyer is in a particularly good mood, then information that works against purchasing a particular product may not be processed efficiently. The degree of relevance also exerts influence. A euphoric mood will not influence your ability to buy a doghouse if you do not own a dog. But your mood may interfere with processing less relevant information. You may purchase an article of clothing when you are in a good mood, and the fact that the item doesn't match other clothing you own may have a low degree of relevance. In a less happy mood, you may be more likely to consider the facts of a buying situation and less likely to allow your emotional state to nudge you into a decision you will later regret. The phrase "buyer's remorse" probably reflects in part the discrepancy between the shopper's mood at the time of purchase and the mood later in the day.

This is not to say that you should shop when you're in a bad mood, but rather that you should be aware that today's shopping environments are designed to lift mood. The lighting, colors, music, and odors are chosen for their ability to influence mood. There is no odor—or other sensory stimulus—which specifically *causes* a person to buy something. But sensory stimuli, including odors, can influence a shopper's mood and therefore affect buying behavior, as evidenced by studies, including our Nike study (see chapter 7) that suggested that in the presence of a pleasant odor, shoppers may assign greater value to a product than they do in an odorless environment.

The context of fragrances may influence shoppers as well. The smell of pine may evoke a nostalgic response, which then makes a shopper more likely to purchase festive holiday decorations for their homes. The aroma of coffee or freshly baked cookies may cause a shopper to think that a cup of coffee and a snack would sure taste good. We always have choices, of course. We can choose to go home and make a pot of coffee or we can head for the cafe that is creating the odor.

Expectancy also influences mood and the ability to concentrate. This is easily seen when you note your attitude toward an event. If you expect to have a good time at tonight's party, you probably will. Your mood will be consistent with the state of positive expectancy. If you expect to do poorly on a history exam, then you are more likely to perform poorly, thereby matching your expectation. Researchers have found that expectation about an event can override the actual experience. When volunteers were told that a research project for which they were asked to volunteer would be fun and a pleasant experience, they had a good time, even when the actual conditions were not particularly pleasant. Of course, we all know people who will stubbornly maintain an negative attitude toward something just so they won't be proved wrong! Expectations shape reality in profound ways.

I Feel Ambitious

In a study that included both men and women in an office environment, it was shown that in the presence of a pleasant odor (five different odorized air fresheners were used), participants set higher work goals and were more likely to work more efficiently than they did when working in an unscented room. In a study involving negotiation, a pleasant odor decreased confrontational behavior and subjects were more likely to make concessions, while at the same time setting higher monetary goals in the outcome of the negotiation.

In some situations, smells are associated with a pleasant experience, and the happy mood that is evoked may have little to do with a physiological response to a specific odor. For example, my daughter Camryn was always very happy when she went to preschool. The classroom at her school always had a strong odor of Play Doh, and Camryn developed a conditioned response to Play Doh, which is a common childhood art and play material. It is possible that if the same odor were added to her other classroom environments, she would feel happy in response to the odor. A conditioned response to an odor is very powerful and has a lasting unconscious effect.

The first experience of an odor and the associated mood have a lasting effect, even if only on the unconscious level. For my daughter, the aroma of Play Doh is associated with an emotionally charged event, her pleasant preschool experience. She will recognize—identify—the odor of Play Doh when she detects it and her memory will include the emotional event. This is one of the reasons that your mood can shift and the content of your thoughts change so drastically in the presence of an odor with which you have emotional associations.

As you can see, adding specific odors to the office, classroom, or home environment may facilitate an alert but relaxed mood or simply lift your mood. An odor will not solve every problem, but common scents may help you focus on your job or on material you need to learn. Odors may also act indirectly to help you solve problems that interfere with performance and learning. Fatigue is one such problem.

Bushed, Drained, Tuckered Out, Drowsy, Sleepy, and Downright Tired

Our language probably has more words and phrases to describe tiredness and fatigue than the Inuit language has for snow. This is not surprising. Many men and women slog through their days in a sleep-deprived state. Consider yourself unusual if you know even one person whose sleep cycles coincide with the daily and seasonal cycles of light and darkness. Most of us need alarm clocks to awaken in the morning because an adequate night's sleep is so rare. We tend to stay up too late, and then, on each tired morning, we resolve to go to bed earlier and get more rest.

Young people also tend to get less sleep than recommended, a fact to which any classroom teacher can attest. Inadequate sleep interferes with both memory and learning, as well as with performance on work-related tasks. Equally important, persistent fatigue can affect mood, which in turn has an impact on memory and learning.

A 1997 survey conducted by the National Sleep Foundation (NSF) measured the "Sleep IQ" of Americans, and according to this foundation, many of us are ignorant about the critical importance of sleep. For example, many people believe that we need less sleep as we age, which is a myth. In addition, most people believe that our bodies adjust to night-shift work, even though it has long been known that third-shift workers report sleep disturbance and are more prone to infections because of lowered immune system functioning.

In their 2001 survey, the NSF reports that the typical adult in the U.S. sleeps seven hours or less on weekdays, while most people need eight hours of sleep in order feel completely rested and alert. About 20 percent of our population report being resigned to the fact that sleepiness will interfere with daily activities. These individuals try to "catch up" on sleep during the weekend. About half of us state that we have trouble falling asleep or staying asleep, that we wake earlier than we need to, or that we do not feel rested in the morning. Depression is linked with sleep disturbance and eight of ten adults suffering from depression report sleeping poorly.

Our work habits influence sleep as well. 40 percent of Americans report working more hours now than they did five years ago; the average adult puts in 46 hours on the job, but 33 percent report working 50 hours or more per week. So, it is not surprising that half of adults in the U.S. say they spend less time in sexual activity than they did five years ago. Adults who work the longest hours report sleeping poorly. In fact, hard-working adults in their twenties report more trouble sleeping than do adults over age sixty-five.

We may associate sleep deprivation with adults spending long hours surfing the World Wide Web, but in fact, less than 25 percent of adults report Internet activity within an hour of going to bed. But adults do report that having something on their minds does interfere with sleep a few nights each week.

Physical problems such as snoring and "restless" leg syndrome interfere with sleep, but these conditions are not necessarily diagnosed and treated. Snoring is a symptom of sleep-disordered breathing and should be treated, so talk to your doctor if snoring interferes with your sleep—or your partner's sleep. Insomnia from any cause should be reported to your doctor, because sleep deprivation can have more ominous implications. Over 50 percent of adults report feeling drowsy while driving, and one in five admit to having dozed off at the wheel. Lack of sleep is a major factor in auto- and work-related accidents, so sleep deprivation should not be written off as just a problem of modern living.

I believe many individuals have been fooled into thinking that after working such long hours, watching late-night television or surfing the Web are relaxing activities—almost as good as sleep. Perhaps because many people are working harder and longer, they don't want to miss what hours they do have available by sleeping. Most of us do not consider sleep a leisure activity. A few decades ago, having a television in the bedroom was almost unheard of, but today, this room is sometimes dominated by an "entertainment" center. I have no doubt that having a television (and computers and exercise equipment) in the bedroom is one of the reasons many individuals have sleep problems. Most sleep therapists — and sex therapists, too — believe that sleep and relationships would improve greatly if the bedroom again became associated with eroticism and sleep. Along these lines, I recommend rearranging your home if at all possible to create a relaxing atmosphere in your bedroom. This is especially important if you have chronic difficulty falling asleep.

Odors, Relaxation, and Sleep

In a number of studies, lavender has been shown to increase alpha wave activity in the brain. Alpha brain waves are associated with relaxation and meditative states. Progressive relaxation exercises, for example, increase alpha wave activity. In a study of insomnia among the elderly, the odor of lavender was found to induce relaxation and sleep, suggesting that lavender may have potential as a treatment for insomnia. As I said earlier, lavender has not been shown to relieve symptoms of anxiety, but not all insomnia is related to an anxious mood state.

If you like the odor of lavender, you can add it to your bedroom environment in several ways. For example, you can burn a lavender-scented candle in the bedroom for a few minutes before retiring. (Remember to put the candle out before getting into bed; it is dangerous to fall asleep with a candle burning.) You can also use lavender-scented sachets in the bedding. You could also buy lavender-scented oil and take a few sniffs in each nostril before getting into bed. Scented eye pillows have become very popular and lavender is one of the most popular scents used. Just place the pillow over your eyes when you get into bed and breathe deeply. If you do not enjoy the odor of lavender then you are unlikely to relax, so this does not apply to you. Since lavender was one of the odors that, when mixed with the scent of pumpkin pie, increased male sexual arousal, you can use it to enhance a romantic bedroom mood as well.

You may have trouble sleeping if you do not prepare yourself to sleep. If you watch a stimulating television movie, complete with shoot-outs, chase scenes, and a range of emotional highs and lows, you may find that you have difficulty drifting off to sleep a few minutes later. Adding a relaxing scent to your living room late in the evening is a good strategy as part of preparation for sleep. The effort is worth your time, because sleep deprivation will affect your memory and ability to learn new information. It is also a lifestyle issue over which you have some control.

Natural or Artificial Odors?

In popular aromatherapy, essential aromatic oils are used in therapeutic "recipes." These oils, derived from the flowers, bark, roots, and leaves of plants, are found in specialty shops and health food markets. Essential oils have a role in plant reproduction and in keeping plants healthy, and from ancient times they have universally been used medicinally, in spiritual and cultural rituals, and to enhance sexual life.

Many of the odors mentioned in this book are available as essential oils. However, it is unnecessary to purchase scents in this way. The artificial—manufactured—counterparts of these odors are equally effective. Every day you are exposed to dozens of artificial odors, from the lemon scent in your laundry soap to the fragrance of sea air in your shower gel.

Consumer studies have shown that these mass-produced odors are often preferred over the natural scents. For example, consumers prefer artificial raspberry odor to the odor of fresh raspberries. The smell of leather in luxury cars is an artificial odor sprayed over the natural leather because consumers like the manufactured scent better. An odorless product is in actuality a product that is scented with a neutral, "no-odor" scent.

The majority of research about odors and their influence on human behavior has been performed using *manufactured* scents. Natural oils are not only prohibitively expensive for research purposes, but these oils are also unstable. The concentration of the odors varies from plant to plant, and even the time of day at which the oil is collected will influence the chemical composition of the oil. So, while these natural oils are pleasant and I don't discourage you from using them in your home or office, the artificial scents are just as good.

In addition, we are still a few years away from true, scientific aromatherapy. While I encourage you to experiment with odors to subtly enhance your memory and ability to learn, I do not recommend that you self-medicate with artificial or natural odors as a substitute for seeking medical counsel, and unless a physician specifically prescribes an essential oil remedy, do not *ingest* essential oils in any form.

Creating Your Odor Library

Most of us have favorite colors, music, textures, and foods, but seldom does anyone ask us about our favorite smells. I invite you to keep track of the influence of odors on your mood. Make conscious choices about your favorite smells the same way you deliberately consider your favorite colors when you purchase clothing or home furnishings. Use the following questions to guide your choices and then keep track of your moods. Your goal is to learn more about your personal response to a variety of scents.

Do you find the floral odor impregnated in the bookmark pleasant, apart from its association with learning? If so, plan to use it for other activities, such as pleasure reading or when you need help concentrating.

What are your favorite holiday odors? Why do they lift your mood? Write down your associations with these odors. Perhaps you can use those holiday smells to alter your mood when you need a boost.

Have you tried new scents lately? I encourage you to experiment with new odors—try a new scent each week and monitor how you feel wearing the fragrance or having it permeate your home.

Do you respond differently to odors depending on the time of day? You may like the woodsy, green smells during the day and the fresh ocean breeze at night. With all the variety available to you today, your odor library may change throughout the day.

Which odors make you feel awake and alert? Jasmine and peppermint, for example, are known to promote a wakeful, alert state. Start with these odors and experiment with others.

Which odors relax you or improve your mood? Responses to odors are individual, so try a wide variety of scents and note your change in mood. Popular individual floral or plant odors, such as rose, lily of the valley, or orange blossom, may or may not influence your mood; the same is true for the common odors such as vanilla or cinnamon. For this reason, I recommend experimenting and monitoring your mood. When you find smells that please you, work them into your lifestyle. Just as you make an effort to listen to your favorite music, give yourself many opportunities to enjoy your favorite scents.

Record all your odor associations. In the coming decades, we will have increasing knowledge about the effects of many odors on mood, learning, memory, and a variety of health issues, such as insomnia and headaches. If you write down your responses to odors, this new information will have greater meaning for you. Consider your "scent impressions" as personal experiments that may or may not match scientific findings.

5

Learn Better, Work Faster

Where there is much desire to learn,
there of necessity will be much arguing,
much writing, many opinions; for opinion
in good men is but knowledge in the making.

– John Milton, 1644

Based on the information presented thus far, you have the
opportunity to enhance your learning and work environments
with the odorized bookmark and with other odors. Although
much remains unknown about the relationship between our
sense of smell and learning and memory, we do know that
odors influence mood, and mood influences learning and
memory. It is up to you to decide if you would like to promote
an awake and alert state as you approach a task, or if inducing a
more relaxed state is preferable. Just because certain odors may
help you work faster, this does not necessarily mean you should
fill your environment with these smells. If an odor is pleasant
and makes you feel better while you work, that represents a
desirable outcome in itself. The goal is to use odors to enrich
your learning and work situations, which may or may not
include working faster, although most of us strive to work and
learn with optimal efficiency.

Thus far, our sense of smell is underused in our educational
system and most work environments. However, this situation is
likely to change in the coming years, as we identify specific applications for odors. In chapter 1, I explained that in our study

using a mixed floral odor, subjects performed a task requiring a wide range of mental abilities (a trail-making subtest of the Halsted-Reitan Test Battery). In the presence of the odor, these individuals performed the task an average of 17 percent faster.

The odor of baked goods or citrus and other pleasant smells did not produce this effect, and we do not know why the floral odor induced subjects to perform so well because we have not yet localized the *neurophysiologic* mechanism that would provide a specific explanation. It is possible that a mixed floral odor had a direct influence on neurotransmitters, many of which are involved in olfaction as well as learning and memory. In fact, there are numerous mechanisms by which neurotransmitters could be involved. For example, it is possible that the floral odor stimulated the release of the neurotransmitter norepinephrine, which in turns stimulates the reticular activating system, a mechanism in the brain that is activated when we feel awake and alert. When the reticular activating system is stimulated, the hormone vasopressin is released. Vasopressin is one of the hormones released in response to stress. In addition, norepinephrine also stimulates the release of the hormone ACTH, which increases attention. Put simply, the chemical responses to the floral odor may have heightened attention and awareness that resulted in faster learning.

The hormonal substances, vasopressin and ACTH, are released in response to both mild and severe stress, and a new learning situation is always mildly stressful. Nowadays, many people hear the word "stress" and have a negative reaction. However, our bodies are always undergoing the stimulation of various types of stressors. The chemical responses to a new learning situation are normal and are not harmful to the body.

While the floral odor is pleasant, most people find the odor of baked goods pleasant, too, but that appealing smell did not produce the same results as the mixed floral scent. It is possible that the floral odor we used in the trail-making test may have both enhanced alertness and decreased anxiety. This test involves left brain functions such as number identification and spatial analysis, and the floral odor may have acted directly on sites in the brain related to these activities.

Anatomically, the olfactory system is part of the limbic brain, the center of emotional life. Positive and negative responses to odors are immediate and occur before the odor is identified. The men and women in our study may have had a positive reaction to the odor, which affected their mood and perhaps even caused a nostalgic response, which generally influences mood in a positive way.

The effect of the odor on performance continued from the second trial to the third, although the effect of the mixed floral scent diminished somewhat on the third trial. This suggests that the study participants adapted to the odor and their perception of its presence became impaired. It is also possible that the mood shift in response to an odor is transient and the subtle lift experienced in the presence of a pleasant odor diminishes over time: the effects of any sensory stimulation diminish over time and the most intense response to sensory stimulation is at the beginning of the experience. A third explanation is that the task itself was too easy, so that after only two re-tries, they reached the maximum speed, given the limitations of time allowed. Had we introduced a more complex test, the learning enhancing effect of the odor may have continued.

Neurotransmitters, Learning, and the Nose

Acetylcholine is another neurotransmitter involved in both olfaction and learning. Phosphatidylcholine, a drug we use to treat those with diminished sense of smell, is known to increase the level of acetylcholine in the central nervous system. In patients deficient in acetylcholine, which includes those with Alzheimer's disease, phosphatidylcholine may improve mental functioning as well as olfactory ability. Likewise, a dopamine agonist, amantadine, may improve olfactory ability and intellectual functioning in patients with Parkinson's disease. Serotonin is another overlapping neurotransmitter, and reduced levels of this chemical are associated with depression. Amitriptyline, a substance used to treat diminished ability to smell, is also used to treat depression, and depression often results in impaired learning and memory.

Finally, it is possible that the floral odor acted on functions that have little to do with intellectual functioning. Perhaps the odor of flowers influences hand-eye coordination or the part of the brain that regulates fine motor movements. To date, there is no evidence that odors affect motor function, but this is a new frontier of research and we cannot rule out the possibility that odors have a direct effect on different brain functions involved in development and learning. I have no doubt that we will eventually determine odors that enhance various kinds of tasks, or, to put it another way, optimal scents for art and music or science and math.

Math and Oranges

A study conducted in Japan found that exposure to certain scents, specifically "citrus green," a citrus and pine combination, and "citrus citrus" (these classifications are used in perfumery) prevented the increase of cortisol, a stress hormone, when college students were asked to do very difficult math problems. This, of course, has implications for ways to control stress in work and school environments, since excessive stress can interfere with learning, recall, and performance.

A large Japanese company diffuses different odors throughout the workplace during the day. In the early morning hours and right after lunch, citrus is used as a stimulating odor. In the late morning and afternoon, floral scents are used because they are thought to improve concentration. During evening hours, woodsy scents such as cedar are introduced. By rotating odors, this company's managers are making broad assumptions about daily cycles of energy and relative states of alertness. This is not unlike what I am suggesting when you keep track of the effect of various odors on your mood state. (See "Condition Your Response" on page 119.)

Would these same odors work in U.S. companies? We can't be sure because there is wide cultural variation in response to odors. For example, the scent of baby powder has a soothing effect on individuals in the U.S. In other cultures, the odor is not associated with childhood and hence no conditioned response to baby powder exists.

Mangos and Limes and Boys and Girls

In 1996, Rajesh Rao, while a high school student in Brookfield, Wisconsin (a suburb of Milwaukee), conducted a study (later submitted to the Westinghouse Science Talent Search) to determine if the classroom environment would be improved by introducing odors. Both students and teachers participated in his study, which was designed to assess four positive mood responses (happiness, energy, concentration, and relaxation) and four negative mood responses (stress, fatigue, confusion, and irritation) to a variety of odors. Rao's study included 137 students and 26 teachers who completed an assessment of six aromas: lime, jasmine, mango, clove, coffee, and sandalwood. (Each odor represents a classification of odor, i.e. sandalwood is woodsy, jasmine is floral, clove is spicy, and so forth.)

Students and staff showed different responses to the odors, and male and female study subjects also showed differences in odor preferences. For example, 58 percent of male teachers but only 43 percent of female teachers thought lime was the preferred ambient odor in the classroom. Male staff reported that lime increased happiness and energy levels, and it decreased fatigue among female staff. Because it decreased concentration and relaxation among the women teachers, mango evoked a negative response. The female staff also responded positively to clove and coffee because it reduced fatigue and confusion.

Among students, 66 percent of boys preferred lime as an ambient odor in the classroom, while only 39 percent of girls agreed. Mango reportedly decreased stress among the boys, increased happiness and energy among the girls, and decreased stress and fatigue among female students. Coffee made the boys less relaxed, but decreased fatigue among the girls. Sandalwood evoked negative responses in both boys and girls. Girls reported that it made them less focused and boys said it made them more confused. Despite the differences among the groups, looked at as a whole, male and female teachers and students consistently rated lime and jasmine as the most pleasant and the preferred ambient aromas for the classroom. In general, the study subjects reported that jasmine and lime had the potential to improve classroom performance. Both scents increased positive mood and decreased negative mood states, both of which are important factors in learning and memory.

Rao concluded that since fragrances have the ability to alter mood, their presence in the classroom has the potential to enhance the learning environment. His research is consistent with other workplace and classroom studies. While no one has yet identified the exact odors that will enhance learning in specific subject areas, evidence is accumulating that the link between odors and learning is a measurable phenomenon—and a vast territory ripe for exploration. At this point, our level of sophistication about odors, memory, learning, and performance is related to what is known about the effect of odors on moods. It is nearly impossible to separate the concept of effective odors in the classroom from the way in which odors influence mood.

Shooting Baskets, Coaching Players

At the time of this writing, our foundation is engaged in two studies involving professional basketball players and coaches. The first study is measuring the effect of odors on three-point shooting. Players practice their three-point shot both in the presence and absence of specific scents. If an odor can improve performance, then it can become a contextual cue and will sharpen kinesthetic memory.

The second study enlisted professional coaches as participants. Anyone who has watched a basketball game knows the kind of stress that coaches endure, particularly on an intermittent basis. The most intense stress may last only a few minutes, or even seconds, but those can be excruciating periods. Stress interferes with mental functioning and may impair a coach's decision-making abilities. Our study introduced different odors (lavender, cucumber, green apple, mixed floral, etc.) in a stressful setting and measured increases or decreases in blood pressure in response to these smells. So far, we have completed this testing with lavender and have found the odor to have no effect on these measures of stress. Theoretically, however, green apple and cucumber should act to reduce stress, since these odors reduce fear associated with claustrophobia. We are continuing to assess these odors to determine potential applications.

The purpose of the study is to determine if an odor that decreases blood pressure, thereby reducing stress, could be useful to a coach during the most stressful situations during a game. The odor itself will then become associated with stress reduction and could become a useful tool to enhance the performance of a coach or anyone else working in high stress situations, such as an attorney in the courtroom, commodities traders, surgeons, or air traffic controllers.

How Odors Influence Mood: Two Theories at Work

Two theories exist to explain the way odors act to shift mood or influence behavior. I call one the *lock and key* theory of odors, which suggests that odors act very much like a specific neurotransmitter, a drug, or an enzyme. In other words, this theory holds that an odor has a specific effect on behavior or emotion. If presented with a certain odor, it should produce a specific emotional response, or, at most, a few emotions. When odors are viewed this way, they become much like medications. If you have a particular problem, you could inhale a specific odor, but inhaling the wrong odor would be ineffective much as taking the wrong medication would not help your condition.

The lock and key theory has been proposed in virtually every book about aromatherapy in which specific odors are recommended for specific health complaints. Aromatherapy applications make sense from this point of view, because the odors then act like a drug — a treatment. An argument supporting the lock and key theory is that odors influence the central nervous system outside our conscious awareness. For instance, in one study, we were able to demonstrate changes in brain wave frequency on the EEG of medical students, using such a low level of odor that the medical students could not even consciously detect the smell. We may be influenced by many odors in the environment but may not be able to pinpoint why our moods shift.

An alternative theory, which I call the *general affective theory of aromatherapy*, holds that an odor experienced as pleasant induces a positive happy mood, and when we are in a happy mood, we do almost everything better, from learning to sleeping. According to this theory, a single odor could exert a multitude of diverse effects, thus affecting virtually everything we do. Certainly, some research supports this idea. Pleasant odors evoke a positive response, while unpleasant odors evoke a negative one. Put another way, a person's mood can change relative to the hedonic (pleasure) value of the odor.

To some aromatherapists, pleasant odors can be considered therapeutic agents. I liken this to a drug such as Valium, which theoretically may be considered useful for virtually all medical conditions because it reduces anxiety and makes conditions such as chronic pain or insomnia less bothersome. If we look at odors in the same way, then any odor that induces a positive mood state would have a positive effect on any disease. But would this extend to other sensory stimuli, too? For example, a lovely landscape or birdsong are sensory stimuli that evoke a pleasant mood. Let's say that *Star Wars* is your favorite movie and you always feel happy while you watch it. Perhaps your headache disappears and you feel relaxed and are able to put negative fears and worries aside. Would we categorize this as "Lucastherapy"? If we believe in the general affective theory of odors, then we accept the implication that any sensory stimulus could be used as a therapy. However, this approach trivializes the definition of therapy.

The general affective theory of aromatherapy does not take into account the context of odors. We respond to a particular smell based on what we expect. Garlic-flavored pasta sauce should smell a particular way. If you inhaled the aroma but it smelled like cinnamon-spiced applesauce you might react negatively, even if you generally think this kind of applesauce smells wonderful. An odor that is contextually appropriate in one situation might be considered totally inappropriate in another. The same odor could produce opposite mood states and opposite effects.

A variation of the general affective theory of aromatherapy is that odors may induce a mood congruent with the demands of the immediate external environment. If you are in a situation that requires an alert state, then introducing an odor induces an awareness of the desired state and you become more alert. If you want to promote a relaxed state, then introducing an odor makes you aware of this. In a sense, introducing a scent acts as an additional stimulus to call attention to the desired mood. The same odor may induce opposite mood states in the same person at different times, which, to follow the comparison with Valium, is the way that some drugs work, too. Valium can reduce anxiety in order to improve concentration when taking a test, or it can reduce concentration when the same person is suffering with insomnia.

Based on what we know about odors and learning, mood states, medical conditions, and so forth, we know that response to any particular scent is at least to a degree unpredictable, with many potential factors entering in. For example, your response to an odor may be different from your partner's reaction based on past experiences with the odor, expectations, context, and conditioned evaluation of its hedonic value. You may associate the odor of horses with pleasant childhood experiences; to your spouse, horses may be just smelly animals.

The conflicting theories about the mechanism of odors in part explains why we often speculate about the reasons why research results occurred. For example, when we discuss the response to the mixed floral scent, we cannot pinpoint the exact reason for the measurable positive results on the speed with which subjects performed a task. This range of possibilities underscores the need for continuing research about the effects of odors in virtually all settings.

Condition Your Response

You may be using your bookmark to help you learn and retain new information. Perhaps an important test is coming up or you need to master a new computer program in order to receive a promotion on your job. Perhaps you are learning material for an important presentation. You are creating a state-dependent learning situation in which you condition your response to the scent. Now, you can add another step: that of reducing your stress during a critical test, demonstration, or presentation.

Beginning 30 days prior to the test situation, do the following:

+ *Choose an odor you like and find relaxing—a common household odor is fine, such as orange, vanilla, lavender, and so forth.*

+ *Have that odor nearby and sniff it while you are relaxing and getting ready for sleep each night. A scented candle, a sachet, an essential oil, or even an orange will do.*

+ *On the day of your test or presentation, have both the floral bookmark and the new relaxation odor with you.*

+ *Use the relaxation odor first in order to induce a relaxed state. Inhale the odor in order to relieve stress. Over a 30-day period, you have conditioned your response to the odor and you will be in a more relaxed mood.*

✦ *Next, inhale the floral bookmark odor, thus recreating your association between the odor and your learning task. You will be in a relaxed state while you recall the material you learned.*

Try other odors from time to time; pair them by using one relaxation odor and one learning odor. These home experiments are meant to be fun. Approach them in the spirit of curiosity and choose the odors you enjoy the most.

6

Desire and Motivation Create Attention

My mind lets go a thousand things,
Like dates of wars and deaths of kings.

– Thomas Baily Aldrich

Regardless of the types of learning or memory we discuss, they all require one essential element: *attention*. We often become frustrated when we don't remember something, but we rarely consider the possibility that it is likely that we don't really know what we think we know. When you forget a name, for example, perhaps you were not paying attention when you first heard the name. The same is true other types of facts, including important information that must be retained for success in a college course or on the job. So the question is: What causes us to pay attention?

I Care, Therefore I Learn and Remember

Motivation is key to retaining new information. You will never improve your memory by using odors or any other memory aid if you lack the motivation to pay attention. This is not meant to sound critical; much of the stimuli we are exposed to every day should be forgotten. You watch a movie for relaxation or read a mystery thriller for fun, and then a day or a month or a year later, you can't remember the names of the characters. There isn't anything wrong with your memory when you forget these names because you never intended to remember them in the first place.

Motivation is essentially an emotional process rather than an intellectual one. For example, Lupe, an employee of the health club I regularly visit, is learning to speak English very quickly. I have made an attempt or two to learn some Spanish, his native language, with no measurable progress. Why is he able to learn so quickly? The answer is simple. He is highly motivated to learn English and I am not sufficiently motivated to put the necessary effort into learning Spanish. His quality of life in this country depends on his ability to speak the dominant language, so he pays attention. His motivation comes from an emotionally based desire to adapt to a new country and its dominant culture. My attempts to learn Spanish are not similarly motivated, but are more like occasional intellectual exercises. Without the emotional component that fuels motivation, I will probably not learn more than a few words of Spanish, and these will be the words I hear often enough to retain.

A college student who must pass an important test to be accepted into a graduate program, for example, will be motivated to learn and retain even incredibly dry information. Career plans might depend on doing well on this test. Obviously, the college student places a high value on learning the necessary material. A person who is lukewarm about getting into the graduate program will likely not do as well on the exam, and his or her studying takes on the quality of a chore.

Something as simple as remembering names at a business networking party depends in part on the value you place on the situation. It is possible that you will remember more names in a business setting than you will at a Saturday evening neighborhood barbecue. You may place a higher value on your business than you do on your social relationships. So a potential client's name is retained, but the new neighbors' names disappear, even if you've had a good time socializing with them. Naturally you're embarrassed when you run into them in the grocery store a few days after the gathering. You may notice that they don't greet you by name either. The memory lapse has been mutual, but neither of you wants to be the first to admit it.

In certain situations, we are conditioned to remember or to forget. For example, my six-year-old son Jack vividly remembers his dreams for months after they occur. Many young children recall their dreams and love to talk about them. However, our culture places a higher value on what we call "objective reality," and eventually most children begin to separate their dream-state fantasy world from what adults value and reinforce. A parent might say, "Enough about the dreams, have you finished your homework?" Before long, children remember only an occasional dream, just like most adults.

In both children and adults, nightmares are usually more vividly recalled than emotionally neutral dreams, although sometimes we repress the memory of these dreams because they are too distressing. Another reason we quickly forget most dreams is that they do not "speak" to us in a language we readily understand. Psychiatrists and philosophers have engaged in numerous attempts to assign meaning to the symbols in our dreams, but dream interpretation is far from an exact science. And most of us are not familiar enough with the landscape of dreams to be sufficiently motivated to recall them.

If you place great importance on remembering dreams, then your recall can gradually improve, provided you are willing to:

✦ *Write about the dreams in a special journal or record them on tape.* Few of us retain the details of a dream unless we record the dream within seconds of waking from it. Dream analysis in psychotherapy usually depends on the patient's willingness to either write the dream in a journal or speak into a tape recorder just after awakening from the dream.

✦ *Pay attention to the sensory details of the dream.* Describe the sounds, shapes, colors, and so forth when you write about your dreams.

✦ *Pick out the elements of the dream that "jump out" when you first remember the dream.* You can write about these elements and ask questions about possible meanings.

✦ *As you fall asleep, tell yourself that you choose to remember your dreams.* Dream recall generally improves over time.

Dreams are also a fascinating area because while dreaming an individual may have sensory experiences they do not have in waking life. For example, an amputee may in a dream have both limbs intact. He or she may walk or run or dance in a way that is no longer physically possible. Likewise, a person who has lost the ability to smell may experience the aroma of flowers or food in a dream.

Dreams also allow us to "be" with a person who has died. For a period of time after my father died, I had dreams about him and, of course, he was alive and well in these images. These dreams were so vivid that it was a shock to awaken and discover that it was only a dream. These particularly realistic dreams about a loved one who is gone usually occur shortly after the person has died. As time passes, we gain the ability to accept the person as a "character" who appears now and again in our dreams.

Motivation Is Compromised by Distraction

No matter how much value we place on remembering certain information, distraction can compromise the motivation. As a high school freshman, I was about to take an important geometry test, for which many of us had studied extensively. We were taking this particular test in the auditorium of the school and as we were about to enter, a fellow student had a seizure. (Most likely he was tired from staying up late to study, which made him vulnerable to epileptic seizure activity in the brain.) Most of the students, I included, had never witnessed anything like this and we were very frightened. In part, this was identification. After all, if it could happen to him, could it also happen to the rest of us? The anxiety reverberated among the classmates, and as a result, we all received lower scores on the tests than expected, based on previous performance on geometry tests.

My experience is an example of the way in which emotionally charged events can interfere with retrieval of recently learned information. In fact, if the event is very important, even long-term memory can be influenced. A friend of mine was once teaching material to a new class of adult students and she forgot many of the details she routinely included in this introductory class session. She did well enough that most of the students did not realize she was confused. Later, when she told a friend what happened, he said, "Well, what did you think was going to happen? Your daughter [a teenager] was just hospitalized last night—no wonder you couldn't concentrate." Indeed! We can think we are on top of things and put on a professional face, but the unconscious mind does not forget significant events. For the most part, my friend could function on "auto-pilot," but her concentration, and hence her performance, was naturally compromised by the distraction of a major event in her life.

Concentration, along with motivation, are key to "laying down the engram" (imprinting a piece of information), as well as retrieving it. Concentration simply means the ability to pay attention to something, be it a mathematical formula we need to learn, a sporting event, a lecture on South American archeology, or our mate's dinner table conversation.

Many adults complain about having difficulty concentrating for long periods of time. They may begin thinking about dinner during work and work during dinner. When they are exercising they feel guilty about not spending time with the kids and when they're spending time with the kids they think they should be working. This inability to focus on the task at hand is usually related to stress and even mild anxiety, often the result of the inability to concentrate. It's a proverbial vicious cycle.

The Noise Culture

Reluctantly, I must deliver bad news to those who have conditioned themselves to working or studying with the radio or television on as background noise. *Any* noise interferes with concentration and learning. Even classical music played at a low volume impairs concentration. Apparently, to absorb information and maintain concentration, a quiet environment is best. This may be difficult to implement in your home because so many children are accustomed to background noise in almost every room in the house. Even many adults turn on a radio or television the minute they walk into the house. In some households there is background noise during most meals and the noise environment continues throughout the evening.

Family therapists, including sex therapists, have questioned the effects of continual distraction on family life and communication between spouses. An additional motivation to consider the noise level in your home and increase the quiet periods is that your children's grades may improve and your own ability to absorb information may increase if you condition yourself to work, study, and relax in a quiet environment. I suggest taking a noise survey in your home and gradually make changes. Here is a way to start:

- How many hours a day do you have the radio or television on?

- Do you turn the television off during meals?

- Do your children turn on music or the television in their rooms? Do they study with background noise?

- Does the noise in the children's room distract you or other members of the family?

- Do outside noises, such as street traffic, machinery, and so forth, distract you?

- When was the last time you had total silence in the house?

- Does silence scare you, at least a little bit?

- Do you believe you need noise in the house? Why? What conditioned that belief?

It's unfortunate but true that some individuals are so accustomed to background distractions that silence feels uncomfortable. Distraction becomes a habit. Our society's environment is quite noisy, so it isn't surprising that background noise is the norm. However, to improve your concentration, wean yourself—and your children—off the "noise culture." Take small steps—turn off the radio or television during meals, and, most certainly, do not have the television on for background noise when no one is watching it. When you are trying to learn anything, concentrate in silence—you'll learn much more efficiently.

Odors and Attention

Odors have a role to play in helping us to focus during certain kinds of activities. In one research project, 48 adults (half men, half women) were given a task that required sustained attention.

Specifically, participants were asked to detect the occasional occurrence of visual signals appearing on a computer screen. The task was designed to simulate the kind of work performed by radar operators or quality control inspectors. In order to compare the effects of two odors, peppermint and muguet (lily of the valley), the subjects performed the visual task for three different intervals, once while exposed to peppermint, once while exposed to muguet, and again when no odor was added to the air. The period of exposure to unscented air served as the control segment of the study. Peppermint was chosen because of its known arousing effects, the tendency to promote an awake and alert state. Muguet was chosen because it has a relaxing effect.

Accuracy in detecting the visual signals was significantly improved in the presence of both odors. The effects of the peppermint odor were predictable because of its stimulant effects. However, the effects of muguet were more surprising, although study participants reported that the visual task was stressful in nature. The relaxing effect of the muguet apparently relieved stress, thereby improving attention and concentration. However, the effect may have been unconscious because the study participants did not report that the odors significantly influenced their perception of stress.

It was also interesting that women performed slightly less accurately than men did under the control conditions of unscented air. The researchers point out that this was not surprising since men tend to perform better on visual-spatial tasks. However, in the presence of the odors, women's performance was about the same as the men's, suggesting that women were more strongly influenced by the odor.

Other research focused on two chemical components of peppermint oil, menthol and menthone, to see if when tested alone either influenced performance on tasks requiring concentration. Menthone, which stimulates the trigeminal nerve, appeared to have a greater effect on performance than menthol. (The trigeminal nerve becomes "irritated" by the odor of ammonia or onions.) This suggests that the "wake up and get going" effect of peppermint is related to mild irritation of the trigeminal nerve that occurs when we smell and taste peppermint.

I suggest you find other odors, in addition to the mixed floral odor of your bookmark, that enhance your ability to concentrate. Experiment and come up with your own "concentration odors." Try the following:

+ Peppermint and jasmine stimulate the part of brain that helps you feel more awake and alert. If you feel drowsy when you are trying to study a dry subject, try these odors.

+ Vanilla is a popular odor and seems to lift mood because people like it. Try burning a vanilla-scented candle when you first start to read difficult material or perform a routine task, such as balancing your checkbook.

+ Bring the outside in—odors from nature may create a pleasant, relaxed mood that enhances your ability to focus on a task. Try sandalwood, rosemary, rose, the "woodsy" scented candles, and citrus odors.

+ If you are tense about the material you want to absorb—perhaps a lot is riding on your ability to learn—then try odors that relax you. Lavender scent is relaxing, even sensuous. It may calm you as you begin; then, if you become sleepy, switch to one of the stimulating odors, such as peppermint or a spicy fragrance.

✦ Use a variety of scents and keep track of how you feel as you use them. Repeat the odor during your next study or work session. You can create your own state-dependent learning situation.

Hypnosis and Focus

While hypnosis is seldom used in everyday life, it is one way to focus attention on specific memories. In a hypnotic state a person may recall experiences, even trivial details, that are consciously forgotten. Concentration and focus characterize a hypnotic state. Distractions are minimal, although a person in a hypnotic state is usually able to become alert and aware of the environment in an emergency. Sometimes the experiences revealed under hypnosis are disturbing and a person has tried to suppress them. But they are stored in what we commonly call the "memory bank" nonetheless.

It is also possible to learn information through hypnosis. Hypnotic suggestion is nothing more than imprinting information, although the person may not remember the specific suggestions introduced. (This explains why hypnosis can be misused in situations in which there is an "agenda" about the type of memory that the hypnotist is trying to elicit.)

Hypnosis is sometimes used for pain control because the subconscious mind receives the suggestion that the discomfort of having a tooth drilled, for example, will not cause pain. When this works well, the subconscious influences the patient and overrides the sensation of pain.

Sodium amytal, a drug that is popularly called "truth serum," is another means by which repressed memories are brought to the surface of consciousness. Even trivial details within an environmental context can be recalled. For the most part, however, neither truth serum nor hypnosis has great practical value in everyday life. Obviously, these tools have limited use and are not available to us when we are trying to recall what we need to buy at the grocery store or when we're playing Trivial Pursuit with friends and need to remember the name of an airport in Paris.

Altering Attention Span

Regardless of motivation and the desire to focus, many adults and children complain about their inability to focus on a task long enough to absorb information. By nature, an infant's attention span is very short. Babies crawling around the floor as they explore the new world of objects are easily distracted. If they head for the electrical socket, we can usually distract them by placing a safer object in front of them. As children mature their attention span lengthens, which is why the time devoted to math or language or geography is extended as they move through grade school and on to high school. As adults, most of us can concentrate for several hours on a project unless we are distracted and our attention is placed elsewhere.

Many educational psychologists — and parents — express increasing concern that we are training children to be easily distracted and, in some cases, actually training them to have a very short attention span. Television, admittedly a valuable teaching tool in many ways, is the major culprit. In the U.S., children spend more time watching television — 28 hours a week or more — than they spend in school learning academic subjects. The average thirty-minute television program has five commercial breaks, so every six minutes attention shifts, which becomes normal to children and, unfortunately, to many adults as well. A six-minute attention span greatly influences learning. By contrast, in Great Britain, a thirty-minute television show is aired without commercial breaks. Logically, the attention span of British children is probably about 30 minutes.

Furthermore, in many school settings, we teach to forget. In reviewing my daughter Marissa's fourth-grade homework, I was amazed how much of it involved review of material learned in the previous grade. A brief period of review is normal, but today, many teachers report that the review takes half to two-thirds of the school year! So, a student with good ability to remember will be bored at least half the year. We are in essence teaching children that it isn't particularly important to remember because it will all be repeated anyway. The message may be subtle, but we are discouraging the development of good memory by reteaching material that was previously presented. Between conditioning short attention span, thanks to television, and conditioning to forget, thanks to lesson plans that make the need to retain information less important, it is no wonder that we do not get the results from our schools we expect.

I Can't Focus for More than Five Minutes

Adults who are concerned about retention and retrieval of information would do well to look at what interferes with their attention span and concentration. A colleague of mine commented that the library seems even more dull than it used to. Perhaps he has this perception because the library is one of the few places designed to minimize distractions. Even the computers are placed in such a way that people reading at tables cannot view the visual images on the screen. In fact, the library seems duller than ever because he is used to being hyperstimulated. It takes effort to create a quiet place, free of the distractions that shorten attention span and influence memory.

The Value of "Trivial Pursuit"

Many of us enjoy playing games that test knowledge and the ability to recall. Of course, it is frustrating when we have a "tip of the tongue" experience and we just can't remember some fact that we think we should know. But for the most part, we enjoy games and puzzles that stimulate the mind.

The truth is, these activities seem light and fun, but they have importance for your ability to focus and on the long-term sharpness of your memory. In chapter 2, I discussed the physical landscape of the brain and described dendrites, a part of the brain cell involved in neuron-to-neuron communication. We have learned that the brain changes and new dendrites form and new connections are made and strengthened. This happens through stimulation, the result of flexing the "mental muscles." Games and intellectual challenges provide active stimulation rather than the passive stimulation of television and the noise that seems to surround us.

Busy Rats Have Bigger Brains

A rat study conducted in the 1960s serves to illustrate the value of focused stimulation. Two sets of rats, raised in a laboratory setting, were provided with different environments. One group of rats had a sensory enriched environment, complete with swings and ladders and various other stimulating toys. They also consorted with each other, so to speak, so these rats had similarly stimulated companions. The other group of rats did not have such a good life. They were provided with a food dish—and nothing else. When the rats died, their brains were analyzed. The stimulated group had bigger brains and twenty percent more dendrite branching. In other words, they did not just *appear* smarter, they *were* smarter.

Subsequent studies with mice confirmed that stimulation may increase the size of the hippocampi, areas of the brain involved in learning and memory. In one study, a group of mice that received sensory "enrichment" had 25 percent more neurons than a second group of mice who spent their days in an environment devoid of stimulating materials and "equipment."

One could say that these studies scientifically demonstrate what common sense tells us: A stimulated brain is a fitter and sharper brain. This kind of research has led to great interest in brain development in young children, specifically prior to age three or so. It is believed that to reach optimal brain development babies must have: loving people who touch them in affectionate ways, stimulating objects to handle, exposure to language, and freedom to physically explore their environment to increase stimulation and develop motor skills. Providing these elements will increase their chances of success in later learning settings. The play that young children engage in is their developmental "work," and therefore it is important to provide a rich sensory environment.

Following our foundation's research with students and the mixed floral odor, I designed a set of simple toys (SmartScents) that provide sensory stimulation for developing infants. These toys are scented with the mixed floral odor, but also provide auditory stimulation, soft textures, and bright colors. We have designed the toys to engage all the senses and attract an infant's attention, at least in part because the mixed floral odor mimics a natural smell. From an evolutionary point of view, the brain is programmed to pay attention to odors in nature, as opposed to scents such as plastic. In addition, a mixed odor is similar to the way odors occur in nature. As discussed in the first chapter, the floral odor increased the speed of learning by 17 percent. Because the odor is pleasant, it has a positive effect on mood and reduces anxiety, which may translate to reducing fussiness in infants.

We also designed the other features of the toys to match the developmental stages of infancy. For example, newborns respond to the odorized wrist rattle that provides constant auditory stimulation. The bright colors provide visual stimulation. The toys for older infants provide the opportunity to manipulate shapes and explore spatial relationships. The added mixed floral scent provides olfactory stimulation in addition to engaging the other senses. (Information about these toys is included in the Products section at the back of the book.)

An Optimal Environment Can Be a Simple Environment

Sometimes parents become confused about what constitutes the optimal developmental environment. We know that it does not mean surrounding a child with rooms filled with *expensive* toys, nor does it mean that it is necessary to watch television programs designed to teach young children while they are entertained. Most children will turn simple household items into toys and are naturally creative if television does not continually distract them.

Brain development can be accomplished equally well in economically humble circumstances as in an opulent environment. The difference is in attitude and in how the people around the young children relate to them. No physical or mental activity is, in the final analysis, insignificant when the brain is developing.

Motivating Ourselves As We Age

At the other end of life, stimulation is important too. In fact, the "use it or lose it" adage is as important as we age as it is in the first two or three years of life. There has been a cultural attitude that the mind slows down as we age, that memory lapses are more frequent, and that we might as well accept this. Although I discuss memory, aging, and the gradual diminishment of the ability to smell in greater detail later, it is important to note that stimulation and motivation are the keys to a sharp mind.

Motivation is important because if we expect that learning will be more difficult and, therefore, it is not worth trying to learn new tasks, then this will be a self-fulfilling prophecy. If we are not motivated to keep exercising the brain, it will atrophy, just like a muscle that we do not exercise. I suggest choosing one subject, hobby, or activity you would like to begin learning or improving. Commit to working on this interest or skill in a concentrated way. (See "In Just Fifteen Minutes a Day" on page 137.) You will be doing your brain a favor.

The Batting Average Genius

In your day-to-day life, you are in charge of what you give attention to, and you probably are motivated to learn and retain information within certain fields. You may be motivated to become a better musician or dancer, or you may need to improve your memory in business or social settings. It is in these settings that you are likely to improve your memory.

Have you ever listened to someone who is a walking sports statistician? This person can recite the batting averages of baseball players who played the game fifty or sixty years ago. Another fan may know who is currently on top of the NBA in every category from rebounds to blocked shots. When I was young, I was motivated to learn information on baseball cards because I wanted to be accepted by other boys in my social group. As an adult I have no such motivation so I do not retain much about popular sporting events of the day. Motivation is the only difference between those who are walking encyclopedias in various fields and those who aren't. We don't retain what doesn't interest us.

Your job is to determine what you truly want to learn and

remember. Most of us spend far too much time fretting about not being able to remember this or that, when the fact is that we don't care about the topic. Exercise your memory muscles and focus on things that are important to you and let go of what you are not motivated to learn and you will find yourself much less dissatisfied with your memory.

In Just Fifteen Minutes a Day

If you spend 15 minutes a day, five days a week, 48 weeks a year, you have *60 hours every year* to learn something new or accomplish a goal that requires concentrated attention. Most people want to accomplish more, but each task looks daunting if viewed as one entity.

In 15 minutes a day you could:

+ Begin learning a foreign language.

+ Relearn and practice the math skills you haven't used since high school.

+ Sharpen your knowledge of geography. You'll soon strike fear in the hearts of your Trivial Pursuit opponents.

+ Improve your vocabulary. In 15 minutes a day, you could learn 25 new words a week, and I for one would not want to play Scrabble with you.

+ Sharpen your writing skills. There are numerous books available with exercises designed to improve your written communication, which may help you in your career.

+ Study material that could help you in your career over the long run.

✦ Read three or four extra books a year, perhaps the books that you have been meaning to read.

✦ Memorize favorite poetry, speeches, or passages from spiritual literature.

You'll have 40 extra hours to learn and improve your skills if you set aside just *10* minutes a day for 48 weeks a year to pursue one of your goals. Of course, *20* minutes a day gives you *80 hours* a year. Or, 33 minutes a day would mean—you do the math!

7

I Remember You

You left three years ago,
Still, your perfume haunts my
solitude. Even now my room is
filled with it, but where are you
my beloved?

— Li Po, *The Absent Lover*

The way human societies are organized and the signs and symbols of status—and the lack of them—cannot be separated from the sense of smell. Throughout history, the sense of smell has played a direct role in defining social class, as well as separating ethnic and racial groups and, by extension, social groups and families. Auguste Galopin, a nineteenth-century physician, speculated that working-class marriages most often take place between men and women with similar jobs because the woman's scent would harmonize with the man's. In that time, particular jobs were associated with odors that workers might carry home with them. So, according to Galopin, the need to harmonize odors logically led to hairdressers marrying perfumers or for the daughters of tanners to marry tanners.

In the early twentieth century, sociologist George Simmel reflected on relations between the classes:

> It may be true that if social interests should dictate,
> many members of the upper classes would be prepared
> to make considerable sacrifices in their personal

comfort and forgo many privileges on behalf of the less fortunate. . . . Indeed, such privations and sacrifices would be accepted far more readily than would any direct contact with the populace, smelling as it does of "the sacred sweat of its brow." The social question is not simply a moral question; it is a question of the sense of smell.

Somerset Maugham expressed this idea a bit more simply when he speculated that the daily morning bath divided people more effectively than birth or education. In our culture, the nearly universal availability of hot water has led to a pre-occupation with personal hygiene, the likes of which has never been seen before. In the past, the wealthy in any culture could cover their body odors with perfumes; today in industrialized nations, almost everyone can scrub themselves clean on a daily basis, and use deodorants and mouthwash, and that's before we even start cosmetic "treatment." We spend considerable time and money covering up natural body smells because intuitively we know that odor impressions become lasting memories and our society tends to be unforgiving of "odor" lapses.

Social Memory Goes Modern

Social memory is an important part of our everyday life, and it involves even more than remembering the names of those we meet in social or business settings, along with other infor-mation about these individuals. Social memory also includes conscious or unconscious impressions we leave on others and others leave on us. Although using odors to help us remember names is possible, and the way I recommend doing it is playful and fun, too, it is equally important to understand how odors influence social and business relationships in subtle ways.

Your Odor Signature

Each person has a unique odor, as unique as a fingerprint. This personal scent is called an odor signature, and it is largely determined by one's genetic profile, or genome. Your odor signature is innate, cannot be changed, and generally is detected on an unconscious level. It is unrelated to added odors, such as colognes or scented shampoos, and also has no connection to personal hygiene.

In the chemistry of attraction, one's odor signature is probably more significant than physical features. A man might say he is attracted to a particular woman because he likes her smile or her figure, but those are reasons that explain an attraction in rational terms. On an unconscious level, the nose is attracted, and then the intellect rationalizes the decision. A woman may believe she finds a man attractive because of his eyes or his hands, but his odor probably attracted her first. His hands and eyes happen to be appealing too, but the sense of smell made the initial connection. The facts about a person that may make him or her a desirable or "appropriate" mate — his or her career, income, race or ethnicity, religion, and so forth — are irrelevant to the nose. When we wonder why a pair of opposites are wildly attracted to each other, we should look to the nose for an explanation.

In social environments, which include the workplace as well as social gatherings, a person's odor signature will play a part in if and how they are remembered. This is essentially an unconscious process and may account for an initial positive or negative impression of another person. In most cases, however, the signature odor does not determine if we will remember the person's name or if we will do business with someone we meet. The odor signature is most powerful in the arena of sexual attraction.

A non-innate type of odor signature is the impression we create with added odors. Obviously, we influence the way we smell by the kinds of scents we use on our bodies and clothing. Depending on the intensity of these scents, they are detected on a conscious level. A person who admires your cologne, for example, is not necessarily attracted to your odor signature, but may respond favorably to the odor impression you have created.

Leaving Lasting Impressions

Perfumes, colognes, and other scented cosmetics are used so commonly in our culture that for many people they are part of daily grooming. Although women are considered the "perfumed" sex, and indeed 94 percent of women regularly use fragrances, 77 percent of men use colognes too. Only 3 percent of women and 8 percent of men *never* use fragrances. Women tend to use scented cosmetic products and colognes more frequently than men do. Men report using colognes in situations involving women, but women tend to use odors because they like them and feel good using them.

In addition to the broad categories of gender and the use of fragrances, social scientists have come up with other systems and labels that define different social behavior. For example, those labeled *high self-monitors* are aware of how others react around them and they attempt (consciously or unconsciously) to control their social image by the odors they use. These individuals may use many different colognes and other fragrances, depending on the setting. Those labeled *low self-monitors* tend to be less aware of other people's perceptions and they use odors to express their own personality. These men and women choose one odor they believe matches their personality and wear it in many different settings.

Men and women who are in a position of leadership or authority, such as teachers or high-level managers, should be mindful of the impact of their odors on others. If they are not already high self-monitors, they should practice high self-monitoring behavior and tailor the odors they wear to the situation and setting. Our fragrances are important features of overall image and contribute to the ways in which we are remembered.

If this sounds superficial, consider that research has confirmed that humans tend to evaluate others in very superficial ways. Entire industries revolve around our preoccupation with physical attractiveness and image, and considerable research shows that individuals considered attractive are liked more than those deemed unattractive. Beyond that, attractive people are also perceived as being more capable than less attractive individuals. Choices in clothing, hairstyles, and even briefcases and watches are often made based on their potential to enhance physical appeal and to project a desired image. Odors form part of the image, and because the sense of smell is so closely linked to emotions, the first odor impression is very important.

The Job Interview—Cologne or No Cologne?

Life would be easier if I could definitively state that wearing particular scents would enhance your professional image. Unfortunately, the evidence isn't so straightforward. For example, in one study, male interviewers gave lower ratings to job applicants who wore colognes than to those who didn't. Women interviewers had the opposite reaction. Female interviewers rated scent-wearing applicants higher on perceptions of intelligence and friendliness; male interviewers rated applicants lower in these same qualities.

In addition, the male interviewers perceived themselves as less effective in their role of interviewer when the applicants wore scents. In other words, self-perception was influenced by the fragrance worn by another person. This again shows the subtle and unconscious power of odors, even in professional settings. The researchers concluded that men were less able than women to ignore unimportant features of a job applicant's grooming or appearance.

What does this mean for your job interviews? If you know that you will be interviewed by a woman, then wearing cologne is probably safe. If you are sure the interviewer is a man, then skip the perfume. In situations where you will be interviewed by more than one individual or you do not know the sex of the interviewer, then play it safe and do not use scents.

Let Me Help You

One element of casual social behavior is helping a stranger in various kinds of non-threatening situations. For example, if a woman is walking down the street and she drops a stack of papers she is carrying, it is likely that a few passersby will stop and help her retrieve them. Likewise, if a man drops a handful of change and it scatters around a phone booth in a public place, others around him will usually pick up the coins and hand them back. Of course, a few people will ignore the event and go on about their business. They may be rushed or in a bad mood or they may not be well developed socially.

It appears that the presence of pleasant odors may influence this type of "helping" social behavior. In one study, researchers staged the need for stranger-to-stranger help in a shopping mall. The study was designed to have an individual ask another person of the same sex for change for a dollar, which is a fairly common stranger-to-stranger request. Another staged opportunity to help involved dropping a pen when a person of the same sex was nearby and, therefore, could easily retrieve it for the stranger. (Apparently, the management of the mall did not want cross-gender requests for help because they could be perceived as "pick-up" attempts, thereby annoying the shoppers. In addition, in our society, even socially gregarious women could be somewhat threatened by requests for help, no matter how polite, from men they do not know.)

Half these requests for help were staged near businesses that had pleasant fragrances surrounding them, such as bakeries and coffee shops and stores where scented candles and other odorized products were sold. The other requests took place near shops that were more odor neutral, such as shoe and clothing stores. Perhaps not surprisingly, passersby were more willing to offer help to a stranger in the presence of the pleasant scents. When these "social helpers" were interviewed after the fact, they reported being aware of the pleasant odors near the coffee stands and bakeries and rated the "odor conditions" higher in these areas. The specific odor did not matter. For example, the same degree of helping behavior and positive response to the odor occurred in the presence of cinnamon rolls as occurred in the presence of coffee or scented candles. Similar results were found in studies that investigated social helping in task-oriented settings. The presence of a pleasant fragrance not only improved performance on these tasks, but evoked more helping behavior as well.

Participants in the shopping mall study also reported that their mood was mildly influenced by the odors. Apparently, the slight lift in mood associated with the pleasant scents resulted in a greater willingness to help a stranger. If positive social behavior can be influenced by odors, think of the implications for society in general, and for interactions within specific institutions such as schools and offices.

Of course, a pleasant fragrance is only one way to evoke a

helping mood. In general, being in a positive mood is the greatest predictor of social helping. Social research has confirmed that giving people a small unexpected gift, such as a bag of candy or a memo pad, will increase their willingness to help others. In another shopping mall study, customers who unexpectedly found a coin in the coin-return slot in a phone booth were more likely to help a stranger pick up a sheaf of papers that were scattered on the floor than those who did not receive this unexpected windfall of a coin. (If it seems odd that a person's mood could lift over such a small event as finding a quarter in a change slot, consider how quickly many of us become irritated over a missed elevator or a driver who is slow to move when the light turns green.)

It Smells Good—It Must Be Worth More

Marketing experts are well aware that odors influence consumer behavior, which is why many millions of dollars are spent to develop scents to make shoppers more conducive to buying particular products. Our foundation conducted a study involving 51 shoppers who were asked to evaluate two pairs of Nike shoes; one pair was placed in an odor-neutral room, the other had a floral aroma filtered into it. Shoppers generally responded more favorably to the shoes in the odorized room, and were willing to spend an average of $10.33 more for them. The simple addition of a pleasant scent added value to the shoes.

Similarly, odors have commercial implications for leisure time activities, too. In our study of gambling behavior in Las Vegas, we added odors to areas in the Las Vegas Hilton casino and measured how much money gamblers were willing to spend based on their location. We assessed gambling behavior in the presence of no odor and then with a pleasant odor added. We found that gamblers spent an average of 45 percent more at a slot machine in the odorized area than at a slot machine with no added scent. Then, when we increased the concentration of the odor, gamblers spent 53 percent more. Although no definitive answer exists that explains why this occurred, we can assume that the pleasant odors altered mood, perhaps making the gamblers more optimistic and ready to spend more money.

How Will You Be Remembered?

Our family and friends, and virtually all the men and women who know us well, retain an overall impression of us, even if they do not see us for a long time. I have a friend who is careless in his appearance and hygiene and always smells bad. I haven't seen him for a year, but I can't think of him without remembering how bad he smells. His smell became a dominant negative feature in my mind, and I cannot will the impression to go away, even when I try to concentrate on his positive qualities.

Sometimes, smelling bad is a conscious choice. Some of the homeless men and women who are mentally ill, specifically those suffering from schizophrenia, may use their bad smell as a device to keep others away from them. They are isolating themselves by choice, even if it is not a healthy choice. When they control their illness with medication and they function more normally, they no longer have the need to smell bad as a way to enforce their desire to maintain an isolated existence.

In a survey of 800 American women, 43 percent indicated that a person's smell was one of two most important personal attributes they noticed when first meeting a person. Face, eyes, and voice were also noted and appear to be dominant features of first impressions. A Japanese study surveyed women about childhood memories and found that the most frequent smells mentioned were common everyday odors as well as the distinctive odor of a mother or grandmother. It is no exaggeration to say that our odor marks us. An important aspect of social memory involves an awareness of how we will be remembered, as well as the impressions we form of others.

Men and Women Perceive Differently

In an earlier book, *Scentsational Sex*, I reported that men tend to find odors associated with males unpleasant, whereas both men and women found female odors more pleasant. The odors men and women exude include a range of potential pheromones, which are subliminal smells, meaning that they are not consciously detected. However, consciously detected odors also influence the impressions that one sex can make on another. Most certainly, they consciously and unconsciously leave a remembered impression.

I was once interviewed by a journalist from *Cosmopolitan* magazine about male odors and female perceptions of these odors. For example, the odors of male genitals, breath, underarms, and feet are considered relatively unpleasant, yet many women perceive that men smell like these odors. Men need to be aware of this perception and, if they want to be remembered positively by women, make sure their "odor impression" is positive.

While the sense of smell diminishes as we age, women's sense of smell tends to be better than men's throughout life. Statistically, men tend to be the older partner, and since olfactory acuity declines with age, women are usually better than men at detecting odors. So, my best advice to men is to listen if their partners tell them that the lingering odor of exercise clothes or socks in the hamper bothers them or if they turn their nose up at the T-shirt they wear to bed. No one chooses to be associated with an unpleasant odor.

The issue of one's personal odor environment extends beyond the sexual arena. Consider the workplace. If managers or supervisors, both male or female, are unaware that they are releasing unpleasant odors into the environment, they may wonder why their training or directions are ineffective. But people tend to learn less and remember less when they are uncomfortable in a person's presence. And remember that an unpleasant odor does not have to be strong to exert a negative influence.

Communicating without Words

We usually assume that words form the cornerstone of human communication, but in fact verbal content comprises only 7 percent of communication modes. About 65 percent of communication is body language; voice quality is about 12 percent. The remaining 16 percent is a mixture of miscellaneous signals, including odors. While not often mentioned as an important element in nonverbal communication, the odor impression is a powerful one.

One part of social memory involves a recognition that we are remembered, consciously or unconsciously, by our scent, just as we form impressions and remember others by their odor. Another part of social memory involves our behavior in social settings, and one area that receives wide attention is the ability to remember names.

The Troublesome Names

From the networking gathering to the cocktail party to the neighborhood barbecue, most of us are concerned about the social skill of remembering names. Unfortunately, concern about remembering names in a social or business setting can detract from our enjoyment of these events.

Peggy and George have been talking for five minutes and the conversation has been quite interesting. Trouble is, she can't remember his name. At some point, she must ask him, or perhaps the host of the party, to repeat his name. George is in the same situation. He doesn't remember Peggy's name and now so much time has passed that he's embarrassed to ask. Both believe they are "bad with names," as if forgetting a name is a character trait or even a learning disability of some kind. In fact, most people complain that they are unable to remember names of individuals they just met, so this is nearly a universal problem.

In our culture, we believe that others will be insulted if we forget their name and must ask to have it repeated, perhaps even more than once. But most people I know are not particularly insulted by this kind of social memory lapse. It doesn't seem important unless it happens several times with the same person. What I am saying is that our social discomfort is probably disproportionate to the reality of the social faux pas.

That said, I offer a few ways to remember names, some of which may be familiar to you. However, using odors to help you recall names, and perhaps other information about an individual, is a new system, one that will both work and be fun. In fact, if you want to break the ice at a party and open up an amusing conversation, just describe the Odorbet.

Introducing the Odorbet

You are probably familiar with the international alphabet used, for example, to avoid confusion and misunderstanding in ship-to-shore communication. A word is assigned to each letter: Alpha stands for A, Bravo for B, Charlie for C, and so forth. The Odorbet works the same way. A specific odor is assigned to each of the twenty-six letters as follows:

a—apple	n—noodles
b—banana	o—orange
c—chocolate	p—peas
d—donut	q—quail
e—egg	r—raspberries
f—flowers	s—spearmint
g—grapes	t—tea
h—horseradish	u—urine
i—ice cream	v—vinegar
j—Jello	w—Worcestershire sauce
k—ketchup	x—Xmas tree
l—lemon	y—yeast
m—mushroom	z—zoo

Flexibility is one benefit of the Odorbet. If for example, you'd rather associate the letter E with eggplant or endive, then go ahead and change it. Or, perhaps you prefer to think of the smell of woods over the odor of Worcestershire sauce or the smell of pears over peas. And as for U, well, there is a relatively new hybrid fruit called ugly fruit, so go ahead and use that word instead of urine, which admittedly is not appealing. Or, if you know what it smells like, use ukelele! (Since the Odorbet is used primarily as a way to remember names, you won't need the letter U much anyway.)

There are two ways to use the Odorbet. First you can asso-ciate the initial letter of the first and last name, in other words, Mark Sachs would be mushroom-spearmint and Jan Coren would be Jello-chocolate. So, when you meet a new person, you can immediately link the name with the Odorbet and once you remember the initials, the name is likely to follow. (See "The Odorbet Lists" on pages 156 and 157.)

In our informal culture, it is more important to remember a first name than a last name. So, if you prefer to concentrate on a person's first name you can use the Odorbet to remember the first two letters of the name. For example, you would remember the name Nicholas by using the Odorbet device, noodles-ice cream. Bob would be remembered with banana-orange.

When I explained the Odorbet to my wife, she wondered if she would begin associating the odors themselves with the individuals. But I pointed out that the Odorbet actually offers the advantage of not requiring associations with an individual. The Odorbet relies only on associations with the letters of the person's name, not with any characteristics of the individual.

Many devices for remembering names rely on attempting to associate a name with a feature of the individual. But this is difficult in most cases. How many short people are actually named Small? How many wealthy people are named Rich? While it is true that names such as Shoemaker or Woodhull or Greenspan are often remembered because of the features embedded in the name, such obvious associations are rare— and becoming more so. Sure, if we happen to speak Spanish, then we have an association for the name Rios. But our culture is so diverse that it would be almost impossible to make associ-ations with so many complex ethnic names.

Now, if we lived in Denmark the issue of names wouldn't be so complex. Three names, Jensen, Hansen, and Nielsen, comprise over 20 percent of the last names in Denmark. In fact, the names ending in "sen" account for 60 percent of the names. You might wonder what the phone book is like, and furthermore, how to know which Lars Nielsen or Hans Anderson is the one you're looking for. The Danes decided to narrow the choices by adding the person's occupation to the phone book listings. Some Danes are changing their names in order to add some variety, but some of their fellow citizens disapprove of that and the debate continues. It's clear that we will never suffer from same-name monotony in this country.

Another problem with looking for associations with names is the diversion factor. If I meet a person named Ralph Brown, I might spend more time thinking about an association for his name than I spend listening to what he is saying to me. I might begin thinking about associations with the color brown rather than focusing on Ralph. With the Odorbet I can simply think raspberries-apple or raspberries-banana, perhaps repeating it once or twice.

It Starts with An Introduction

Your memory for names—or for anything else you want to learn at a social or business function—will improve if you arrive at the gathering refreshed. If you are hungry, eat something. Fatigue interferes with retrieval and with learning new information, and low blood sugar will deprive the brain of the energy it needs to function properly.

Assuming you are alert and can concentrate, decide if you are truly motivated to remember the names of those to whom you are introduced. Is this learning opportunity of sufficient value to you that you will put your attention to the task? Attention and motivation are critical in social situations because there are usually many distractions. In fact, one reason we forget so

many names is that the process of moving the names from immediate, or working memory, to long-term storage is interrupted.

The following three steps are guaranteed to help:

1. Repeat the person's name two or three times to your-
    self, and assign the Odorbet designations. (This is
    similar to the frequent repetition of names that occurs
    at the beginning of movies and television programs:
    the repetition helps you retain the characters' names
    early in the action.)

2. Repeat the person's name in a sentence, perhaps by
    asking a question in which you use the person's name,
    which gives you an opportunity to say it out loud.

3. If possible, form a visual image in your mind of the
    person and the name. For example, you might note
    that Marshall is wearing a very loud tie or that June is
    wearing red. Or, you can picture the name written on
    a nametag. You might try using your index finger to
    write the name in the palm of your hand

If, however, you find that forming a visual image is distracting
you from the conversation, then skip that step. Just use the
Odorbet technique and repeat the person's name outloud in
your conversation. And relax. In many networking gatherings
and even social events, people exchange business cards and they
are wearing nametags, which reduce the whole problem in the
first place.

This Person Smells Like. . . .

It may seem logical to try to associate the actual smell of a
person with his or her name. In theory, this could work if the
person's name is Rose or April or Grassly or Barnstable. You

can then associate the smell of the flower, a fresh spring rain, freshly mown grass, or stables with the person. If an individual is wearing a cologne that you are familiar with, then you can associate him or her with that fragrance. But in our culture, it is considered rude to sniff a person to detect his or her odor! (In some cultures, sniffing is part of social greeting.) If an odor association comes easily, then use it. But if it distracts you from meaningful conversation, then do not try it.

They're Putty in Your Hands

For our daughter Marissa's fifth birthday, we had a puppet show and a character, Cinderella, who played games with the children. I was amazed that within a few minutes, the puppeteer and Cinderella had memorized the names of all twenty children. When the party was over, I asked these party professionals about their memory for names. They explained that if they quickly learn the names of the children at these parties, they have better control over the group. It's their way of drawing the audience in, particularly the more rambunctious boys. Being able to call the children by name encouraged one-on-one communication, even in the midst of a crowd.

Adults can benefit from this information, and professionals who manage groups or facilitate large meetings understand that being called by name is a form of social bonding. If you remember a person's name and use it often in conversation, your ability to influence that individual increases.

It's Time for a Rhyme

One of my favorite *Seinfeld* episodes involves Jerry's encounter with a woman with whom he quickly becomes intimate. He has a problem, though—he can't remember her name. In a conversation with her, he casually brings up the issue of names, and she mentions that her name rhymes with a body part. So, throughout the episode poor Jerry attempts to recall her name by rhyming body parts. He calls her "Mulva" and "Regina," both of which are wrong of course. She finally leaves him in disgust because he can't remember her name, and then, after she's left and is walking away, he remembers her name and calls after her, "Goodbye, Delores." Such are the problems with using rhymes to recall names. Jerry should have used the Odorbet— donut-orange, no problem!

Using the Odorbet

Test the Odorbet in the following way. Read the following list of names once; study them for a minute or two. *Do not use the Odorbet code.* Then take a separate sheet of paper and write down all the names you recall. Simply count the number.

Then turn the page and as you read them, associate the Odorbet code written next to it. Study the list for a minute or two (the same amount of time you devoted to list #1). Take a separate sheet of paper and write down the number of names you recall. You may be surprised by how many more you can recall when you use the Odorbet.

List 1 (No Odorbet)

Evan Letourneau	Virginia McCullough
Carl Wahlstrom	Renee Mehlinger
Irving Barr	Stanley Block
Robert Egel	George Grodek
Pat Arbor	Marybeth Shean

List 2 (Use the Odorbet)

Richard Doty, raspberry-donut

Kristine Strodthoff, ketchup-spearmint

Steven Schwarzback, spearmint-spearmint

Jan Fawcett, Jello-flowers

Mark Schwartz, mushroom-spearmint

Jim Stern, Jello-spearmint

Rick Bowen, raspberry-banana

June Kaiser, Jello-ketchup

Joseph O'Grady, Jello-orange

Mark Coe, mushroom-chocolate

8

Forgetting Can Be Normal Too

Memory is the thing you forget with.

— Alexander Chase

Rocco is convinced that at least 60 people attended the company cocktail party hosted by his boss, but Jackie is sure that no more than 30 people showed up. Rocco also would stake his life on the fact that the party was held in late summer, but Jackie is equally sure that the leaves on the maple tree were turning red, so it was obviously held in the fall. Each can't understand how the other could have such a poor memory about this event.

Most of us occasionally become frustrated with others and ourselves over memory lapses. It's a common human experience. Now and then everyone is forced to say, "I'll never forget what's his name." You probably become even more frustrated when a fact about which you are absolutely certain is disputed by a person who is convinced "it didn't happen that way." But everyone's memory is quite fallible, so fallible in fact that some of the things you claim to remember may never have happened! On the other hand, you may have no memory of events that others are sure you took part in. You may have heard colorful stories about some childhood antic so many times you don't know if you actually remember these episodes or if you have formed a picture in your mind based on what others have told you. This "visualized" memory then seems much like other autobiographical memories. When it comes to accuracy, childhood memories are among the most difficult to evaluate.

First Memories Are a Special Case

When you think about childhood memories, it often seems that you recall an event here and there or a particular scene, but long periods may be missing. Most people do not remember the process of learning to read, which presumably happened after the age when memories imprint. Infants learn many skills, but virtually no one remembers learning to roll over or sit up. Learning to walk is a complex developmental task involving motor coordination and balance—and considerable trial and error—yet you do not recall the process. Babies and toddlers also learn language and they develop spatial and geographic memory, but virtually no memory traces remain of the first eighteen months to two years of life, the time when the most motor and language skills develop. Even after age two, very few memories exist of ages three or four. Freud called this nearly universal phenomenon "childhood amnesia." Most of us remember almost nothing until around the time we start school.

During these early years, we learn the "scripts" that integrate into daily life in our particular environment. The routines and familiar events of early life are for the most part not recalled, and even later in life we may have only a few dominant memories of events each year. We do not even attempt to remember what we had for dinner on a particular evening of 1976, but we may recall some vivid details about the new job we had that year. Those with a flashbulb memory of the Kennedy assassination usually remember little else about 1963.

At one time, it was assumed that the reason we do not remember events prior to age eighteen months or even later is related to brain development. However, it now appears that the capacity for autobiographical memory is a function of psychological rather than physiological development. The theory holds that autobiographical memory cannot begin until the concept of self is in place. Infants do not see themselves as separate from their parents or others who care for them. To infants, everything in the environment is an extension of them. Between eighteen months and two years, babies begin to understand the difference between themselves and others, at which point autobiographical memories are possible. As we mature, our capacity to develop a sense of self strengthens, and our autobiographical memory begins to take form.

We also can surmise that childhood memories tend to be selective because we choose memories congruent with our adult self-concept. Adults who consider themselves happy and well-adjusted recall happier childhood memories than those who currently are experiencing difficulties. One study of elderly individuals showed that the quality of early recollections can change over time. For example, prior to entering nursing homes or other institutions, men and women recalled happier early memories than those remembered after admission to care centers or hospitals. Their current situation had negatively influenced their recall of the past.

In psychotherapy, the very first memory may become significant in exploring childhood issues. Why do you remember sitting on a chair in your grandmother's house or falling down on the sidewalk after your older sister pushed you? As therapy continues, first memories may change, however, and the new memory may reveal other information to explore in therapy.

I believe that early odor memories are an unexplored area of childhood that could provide insights into the dominant memories that shape current difficulties. Given what we know about odors and nostalgia, it is possible that associations with scents can tell us much about ourselves and the emotional tone of a variety of events in our lives. Even a relatively unpleasant odor can arouse nostalgia, a bittersweet feeling, about a person or place. For example, the odor of horses may be repugnant to most people, but arouse nostalgia among those for whom horseback riding was a favorite childhood activity.

You Are a Hero in Your Own Story

Throughout life, autobiographical memory shifts between the "facts" and the subjective quality of the feelings surrounding events and experiences. For the most part, you dominate your memories, or, put another way, you are the main character in your memories. This is logical, of course. What is autobiography if not your life story told through your personal impressions and experiences? Remembering that each person is his or her own main character helps explain why you and even your closest family members and friends may have entirely different recollections of the same events. Technically, the events were *not* the same because no two individuals have identical experiences.

The past invariably influences current observations, and differing sensory impressions create unique experiences for each person. A person who is unable to smell will not have the same memories of a Thanksgiving dinner as those for whom the aromas represent an integral part of the pleasure of the day. Likewise, memories of past Thanksgivings influence the experience of a current one, which may or may not be remembered later in life. Can you recall every Thanksgiving past age six or so? Probably not, but you have general Thanksgiving impressions and perhaps a few stand out. The first holiday after a birth or a death in the family provides a marker of sorts, a special reason to remember other events taking place that year.

The Way We Were

A natural tendency exists to remember our own actions in the best light possible, and the image of others may suffer by contrast. We also tend to recall ourselves as the dominant person in an event if it improves our image, and vice versa. If police officers apprehend Mary Kay and Diane as they are breaking into the neighbor's house, Mary Kay will probably recall that Diane masterminded the robbery. Diane will likely tell the police that Mary Kay first brought up the idea. In all likelihood, each steadfastly remains convinced about her innocent bystander role in the whole sordid mess.

Criminals offer an obvious example of a universal desire to create a positive view of our role in our life story. If we must create a few scapegoats to paint our rosy scenario, then so be it. How many individuals admit they caused an auto accident or own up to starting an argument? Sometimes, forgetting information supports our best interests!

Hindsight Bias

If you are convinced that you were age twenty-four on your first trip to Paris and later come upon proof that you were actually twenty-six, you are likely to, in hindsight, claim that you weren't all that certain in the first place. Conversely, if you are lukewarm in your conviction about a fact and it later turns out to be true, you are likely to exaggerate your earlier conviction. Apparently, we just don't like being wrong and we will alter the past if necessary to preserve the image of being right— or even almost right.

We see another example of hindsight bias when journalists interview the neighbors of a person accused of committing a crime. From what the neighbors tell us, this man, let's call him James, was a "loner" and at the very least appeared or acted "different" and, frankly, "weird." For months or years, these same neighbors might have described James as quiet or reserved, a person who enjoyed and protected his privacy, but usually behaved pleasantly enough. Now, when he stands accused of murdering a dozen people, neighbors and acquaintances claim they always sensed something seemed quite suspicious about him—and that a gun collection that reporters are talking about always did bother them.

Burying Memories

Sigmund Freud suggested that everything we experience, every sensory stimulus, is recorded and remembered, and therefore forgetting something is a meaningful sign of internal conflict. This hypothesis remains in dispute, but no one argues the existence of different kinds of memory lapses or even memory distortion. Freud described two ways of forgetting: *unterdruckung*, which is suppression, and *vendrangung*, which literally means ousting, but in psychiatric language we call vendrangung the *repression* of memories.

When we suppress a memory, we consciously decide not to deal with the issue at the present time. In essence, we deliberately procrastinate about our worries or concerns. We all do this from time to time. We may say such things as, "I can't worry about the house payment today because I must cope with my sick child," or, "I can't deal with how bad I feel about the fight with my wife because my flight leaves in an hour and I'm running late." Rebecca Rupp, author of *Committed to Memory*, likened this to Scarlett O'Hara's famous words, spoken after the dashing Rhett Butler leaves her: "*I won't think about it today. . . . I'll go crazy if I think about losing him now. I'll think it about tomorrow, at Tara.*" So, we could call suppression the "Scarlett O'Hara syndrome."

On the other hand, when we repress, we attempt to completely forget, to banish a memory completely and bury it so deeply it disappears forever. Presumably, repressed memories are so painful that the psyche cannot handle them and in effect declares: "There will never be a time to deal with this, so I will wipe it out of my memory." Repressed memory has become a controversial issue in recent years primarily because of legal cases filed after individuals claimed to have recovered once-buried memories. Generally, individuals who believe they were sexually abused as children bring these charges. Because of the traumatic nature of the childhood events, the individuals repressed the memories. In adulthood, either specific incidents triggered spontaneous recall or the memories returned during the process of psychotherapy.

The phenomenon of repressed memories probably exists, although many questions remain about the efficacy of considering the recovered memories accurate, particularly long after the alleged events have taken place. Some psychotherapists believe that memories recovered prior to beginning psychotherapy may be less suspect than those recalled once treatment has begun. The American Medical Association (AMA) also agrees that there is a danger of misapplication in using recovered memories to settle legal questions.

The concern involves the potential for patients in therapy to be susceptible to suggestion by the therapist. Memories recalled during hypnosis may be even more inaccurate, because memories can quite literally be created by suggestion, not just recalled.

Psychologists who question the efficacy of long-recovered memory do not question the fact of child abuse. However, the complete repression of all such events is still open to question. Many victims of early abuse remember the experiences quite well and may spend a lifetime trying to forget the traumatic episodes. It is possible that a single terrifying event is more likely remembered than a pattern of repeated abuse. For example, the 26 children that were kidnapped in Chowchilla, California, in

1976 and held in a truck trailer that was buried in a quarry remembered the event after they were rescued and could report details later that proved fairly accurate. Even five years later they still had clear recall. However, these memories may have remained intact because of the group effect and because the trauma to which they were subjected was initiated by a stranger rather than by a person with whom they had an emotional bond and thus had less conflicting feelings toward.

Another problem with recovery of long-repressed memories involves the inaccuracy of most personal memories. We do not know if the traumatic memory recalled is a specific memory of an event or rather is an integrated memory, a representation that has formed from any number of related events. For example, a war veteran may detect the odor of burning gasoline or diesel fuel and this triggers a traumatic battlefield memory. We cannot be certain if this memory is an actual re-creation of an event or a "picture" based on many incidents that are now integrated into one memory.

Most psychotherapists agree that an individual who has experienced the physical and emotional trauma of repeated sexual abuse, for example, is unlikely to have repressed all the episodes. In addition, the mind is so suggestible that therapists can plant the seed of possible sexual abuse and cases have been reported in which the accused person begins to "recall" memories of events that never occurred.

Young children are particularly vulnerable to suggestion. Many reported cases of abuse in daycare centers and preschools, some of which included detailed reports of such things as satanic rituals and bestiality, never occurred. Rather, these reported memories were the consequence of a kind of mass suggestion, in which adults were so convinced that abuse had taken place that the children created memories to "please" the adults.

The Brain May Decide

Clinically anxious patients may or may not be able to link their anxiety to memories of traumatic events. This complicates the issue of repressed memories because recent brain research suggests that stressful events can cause malfunction of the mechanism involved in laying down a memory. Specifically, hippocampal function may be impaired, which may result from the high level of steroid hormones released by the adrenal glands during stressful episodes. The same steroid hormones that allow us to respond to situations in which we must fight or flee may cause damage to hippocampal neurons.

Situations in which severe stress can keep a memory from forming or cause the memory to be weak or fragmented are not the same as those in which stress increases memory and even provides a "performance edge." It is possible that a rapid release of adrenal hormones is responsible for the formation of a "flashbulb" memory. Mild stress is beneficial when taking a test. Severe stress, however, similar to that experienced in abusive, violent relationships or the emotionally traumatic events that occur in battlefield conditions, put one at risk for impaired memory due to changes in the brain. In fact, victims of prolonged abuse and post-traumatic stress disorder (PSTD) may experience shrinkage of the hippocampi. These individuals may show memory impairment, but without any diminishment of intelligence. Animal studies confirm that dendrites may even shrivel under stressful conditions.

The amygdala, a part of brain involved in emotional response, may be conditioned to respond to stimuli, even in the absence of conscious memory of the traumatic event. This may explain what happens when reasons for anxiety are unknown, but the feeling is real nonetheless. No memory can be retrieved to explain the anxious state because no memory is stored. The stress was so severe that stress hormones effectively blocked the hippocampi from doing their job of "indexing" and storing the memory. However, the emotional part of the brain *does* remember and reacts anyway.

Aside from physiological changes in the brain, we know that memories tend to be easily changeable and details are added and altered, often based on simple suggestion. Numerous experiments have shown that memories are not reliable when it comes to personal experiences and even observed events.

Inaccurate Memories/Enhanced Memories

A story is told about a German law professor whose classroom was disrupted when a violent argument broke out between two students. The argument escalated and one student pulled out a revolver and shot the other man. At this point, the professor told his students to write down everything they remembered about the incident. Later, the purpose of the episode became clear when the professor revealed that the fight had been staged. The students' accounts of the events varied widely and most included objectively inaccurate details. Perhaps more valuable than numerous lectures and dry statistics, this exercise provided law students with direct experience about the unreliable nature of eyewitness testimony.

Despite its great potential for error, our courts routinely use eyewitness testimony. Among those who are wrongly convicted, at least half were sent to prison in the first place based on inaccurate accounts provided by eyewitnesses. Considerable research has confirmed that eyewitnesses are susceptible to their own errors of observation, and in addition, they can be easily influenced by suggestion.

Elizabeth Loftus of the University of Washington began studying the accuracy and permanency of memory in the 1970s.

In a study that has now become well known among psychologists, she showed students slides of an automobile accident and later tested their recall of the details. On the whole, their recall was fairly accurate. However, when questions were asked about items, such as traffic signs and cars not originally pictured, the accuracy of the recall began to decline. The students formed answers based on extraneous information and later expressed certainty about the later material suggested and not shown in the slides.

Through subsequent studies, Dr. Loftus concluded that eyewitnesses are not only open to suggestion, they can report such basic information as race and gender inaccurately. Rather than viewing a memory of an observation as a concrete bit of information, it is clear that some memories more closely resemble kaleidoscope images that change with time, especially with the addition of other bits of information.

Researchers who have examined police interviews note the frequent use of suggestion, not necessarily for the purpose of misleading eyewitnesses, but with the same effect. This principle operates when physicians, psychologists, historians, and sociologists question individuals to elicit information. Medical histories, for example, are often inaccurate. Patients sometimes successfully repress information about unpleasant illnesses, and even past surgeries may be left out of patient narratives.

It Never Happened, but I Remember It Anyway

Mark Twain once said: "It isn't so astonishing, the number of the things I can remember, as the number of things I can remember that aren't so." Mark Twain didn't know it, but *cryptomnesia* is a name for this kind of "memory." Cryptomnesia goes beyond the tendency to influence or distort memory. We may, for example, take a story someone told us and turn it into an experience of our own. Apparently, this situation is neither unusual nor difficult to produce.

A group of five-year-olds were once asked if they had ever had five different experiences, of which four were events or incidents familiar to the children. Researchers recorded the children's answers and the questions were repeated weekly. By the eleventh week, one-third of the children claimed not only to have had the fifth experience, but also were providing details about it.

The famous Swiss psychologist, Jean Piaget, told a dramatic example of a cryptomnesic memory. For many years he had a vivid memory of being kidnapped, snatched from his baby carriage on a street in Paris. A toddler at the time the incident supposedly took place, Piaget had a detailed memory of the kidnapping and he recalled his nurse bravely fighting off the attacker. He also recalled the arrival of a police officer that saved him from being carried off by a stranger. When Piaget was a teenager, however, his former nanny wrote a letter to the family confessing that she had made up the story in order to impress her employers. The attempted kidnapping had never occurred, so Piaget created the memory from the often-repeated story.

June, a patient of mine, says she has a memory of sitting on the top of a counter in a butcher shop where her father had left her while he did the family's shopping. Oddly enough, her sister has the same memory. All they know is that her father left one of the two girls in the butcher shop and went home with the groceries. While walking home, he suddenly remembered he'd left his daughter behind and rushed back to get her—she was still sitting there waiting for him. So, which sister was left behind? Which sister's memory is real? Neither parent can remember for sure, so the mystery continues. Over the years, my patient has questioned the detailed picture she has in her mind of the counter in the butcher shop and the image of her father coming through the door to "retrieve" her. Meanwhile, her sister is no longer sure about the event either. Their dad only remembered the terrible feeling he had as he rushed back to the store. The girls' mother remembers only being relieved that the daughter, whoever it was, hadn't wandered away. So, here is a family story that might as well be a scene in a novel. Many childhood memories likely have a cryptomnesic component.

I Know It Hurt, but I Can't Quite Remember It

Pain is a special case because it does not appear to produce significant memories—at least for humans. True, we remember we experienced pain, but for the most part forget the pain itself. For our species, with the capacity to make choices and plan future events, this represents a significant capacity. Usually, pregnancy brings its share of discomforts and childbirth is generally painful. If women remembered the sensation of the pain, we would be a world of mostly one-child families and one can only guess how sexual practices would have evolved in human culture. Most likely, our species would have gone the way of the dinosaur long ago. Over time, the memory of childbirth subsides, making many women willing to go through a pregnancy and give birth again — perhaps many times. This isn't an example of denial, because a woman will remember the reality of true discomfort. However, the memory of the sensation of pain tends not to persist.

The ability to forget pain is probably a built-in adaptive mechanism of the human species. Rats, for example, have a better ability to recall pain. They are conditioned to remember the pain of becoming ill from eating poison, and if they did not remember this pain they would eat poison again and again until they finally died.

Humans do have a conditioned response to familiar discomfort, which is called *somasthetic memory*. If we feel a pain in our knees after jogging on concrete, we change our pattern and jog on cinder or grass. If we didn't recall the discomfort, we would make the same mistake again and again.

There are times when we remember discomfort resulting from an experience, but our relatively poor memory for pain allows us to repeat the experience anyway. Year after year we overeat at holiday dinners, all the while knowing we will be uncomfortable. Or, we may know a certain food gives us heartburn, but we like the food so we eat now and regret later. These decisions are usually trade-offs. Most of us won't risk seriously injuring our knees, for example, but we will risk an evening of discomfort for the immediate gratification of eating a favorite food. Our action does not display our superior intelligence, but the intellect does not rule over pain memories.

Another reason the intensity of pain and discomfort is poorly recalled is related to the strong tendency to alter memories and make them more acceptable, or at least less troubling. Even pessimists tend to put on rose-colored glasses when thinking about the past. It sometimes takes effort to face painful memories because of this natural response to avoid emotional discomfort.

Forgetting Is Part of Our Nature

Important events in your life serve as defining landmarks in the flow of your life. Seemingly minor or trivial memories probably reflect the emotional tone of different periods in your life and provide an overall impression of what is important to you. Imagine what it would be like to remember every detail of each day of 1986 or 1991. You would constantly be flooded with information not remotely relevant to your life today. The fact that the past often seems like a blur of events and impressions, some of which have importance and some of which do not, appears to be a natural part of the human condition. While it is fine to attempt to improve your memory, you should also realize the significance of your ability to forget.

So, Who's Right?

We all have distinct childhood memories, usually something so vivid that we are certain of every detail, including the time of day (perhaps the exact hour), place, participants, and so forth. Choose one of these memories from your early life and write down as much detail as you recall. This could be a special holiday, a memorable incident at school, an accident in your childhood home, a sporting event, an incident occurring during a family vacation, or the day something important happened to your family (a new job, a job loss, a parent's illness, graduation day, a birthday, a family celebration, and so forth).

+ Your age

+ Location

+ Time of day or exact hour

+ Others involved

+ Describe the "special" incident

+ Sensory details (weather, clothing, odors, sounds, and so forth)

+ Emotional details (how did you feel and why did you react with fear, surprise, joy, anxiety, and so forth?)

+ Why is this incident so important to you?

Now that you have recorded all the details you can recall, ask other participants what they remember about the event. Compare notes and see which details match and which do not. Discuss the reasons you believe your version of the event is correct. You may find that each participant remembers an event a certain way because of the variety of subjective meaning attached to it. Your siblings are not likely to have vivid memories of your birthday parties unless something significant happened during the event that made it stand out.

Even intimately shared experiences may be remembered differently because of associations with other "memory markers" surrounding the event. For example, you may say, "I know the accident happened on a Monday because the day before I performed in my first dance recital. It was morning because just before it happened I was hungry and wondering when we would stop for lunch." Another participant might say, "I'm *certain* it happened on a Tuesday because I was nervous about the test I was supposed to take on Wednesday. It had to be evening because I remember it got dark while we waited for the tow truck."

So, who's right? Most of the time we will never find out. Try this with classmates at a high school reunion or ask childhood friends about their memory of an event that is vivid to you. The more we learn about memory, the less likely we are to insist that our version of events is absolutely the correct one.

9

The Trouble with Bad Odors

I have often noticed that
they [odors] make a change in me
and work upon my spirit according
to their properties.

— Michel de Montaigne

The English language—and other languages too—contain numerous words to describe unpleasant smells. Odors we don't like and avoid are called foul, putrid, sour, sickening, or merely bad or unpleasant. Our language reflects the way bad smells are so often associated with negative events or situations. We speak of the "smell of danger," or we say, "He raised a big stink," or, "This situation smells to high heaven"—or just plain "stinks." When we are suspicious about something we may say, "I smell a rat."

When Western religions tell us that heaven smells sweet and hell is filled with a sulfurous stench, they proclaim an immutable link between bad smells and evil, as well as a link between pleasant smells and goodness. This link has had a long history in the development of our language and perceptions, and it continues today. For example, many Europeans were convinced that the Black Plague of the Middle Ages was caused by bad *smells*. There was a strong belief at the time that God had sent the stench of illness to punish human beings for their sinful behavior. Foul odors, also called *effluvium,* were believed to be a primary cause of illness and people went to extreme lengths to protect themselves from air that was polluted with bad odors. Physicians wore elaborate olfactory masks so they would not inhale the odors. During this time, goats became pets and were brought in the house, in part because they smell bad and would help protect the family from disease. This turned out to be less nonsensical than it sounds because in the modern era, scientists discovered a substance in goat urine that is toxic to the bacteria that carry bubonic plague.

The belief that odors can not only cause illness, but are the vehicles by which disease is spread, led to the connection between epidemics and foul smells. Today, we speak with scientific authority about airborne infections, but it is not a new notion. The ancient Greeks and Romans came up with a version of airborne germs when they speculated about changes in the atmosphere that affected the integrity of the air we breath. This "breakdown" in the element of air manifested in diseases and other natural disturbances. The Roman philosopher Seneca believed that lightning was dangerous because it contained a smell that caused pestilence.

During the plague years, many people were afraid to let others enter their homes, because those persons were sure to have been exposed to the bad smell that caused the illness. Some people began using pleasant and, therefore, good or even holy odors to combat the danger of foul smells. Those who were not ill used perfume, herbs, and other strong-smelling substances to protect themselves from the smell of pestilence that hovered all around them. These "good" odors were used in ritualistic ceremonies to ward off the deadly breath of those stricken with the illness, whose origins were linked with evil and God's wrath. On the other hand, some believed that bad odors would protect them from being exposed to disease and these individuals thought it foolhardy to take a bath and wash way their aromatic "armor."

During the medieval period some people thought it was spiritually superior, as well as better for their health, never to wash at all. These individuals believed that they must always appear in a completely natural state before God—dirt, smells, and all. In fact, those who washed were under suspicion for being messengers of the devil. Legend has it that St. Agnes, who was executed and became a Christian martyr at the age of 13, never took a bath because she did not want to mar her purity; others apparently never washed their faces so as not to disturb the holy waters of baptism.

Paradoxically, the populace was also led to believe that witches, warlocks, and heretics exuded a bad smell and, therefore, it was easy to make accusations that were difficult to combat with logic and reason. Since unpleasant odors themselves were thought to harbor evil, it seemed rational to believe that unseen forces that turned them into witches or heretics had touched one's neighbors and friends. By contrast, good smells were associated with holiness. It's no accident that the rose is symbolic of the Virgin Mary and that certain saints were said to smell sweet even after death.

Emmanuel Swedenborg, the Swedish scientist and theologian, claimed that each person exudes a spiritual odor. A greedy person, for example, smells like mice; cruel and vengeful people smell like cadavers. Furthermore, evil doers love bad smells and can't stand to be around pleasant odors. Swedenborg's ideas may sound strange today, but he also believed that freshly baked bread smelled heavenly, so he may have been right after all.

While we know today that pleasant odors can't be categorized as morally righteous and unpleasant odors as evil or profane, our ancestors weren't completely wrong about odors and their connection to illness—or even to behavior. This doesn't mean, of course, that we can call people witches or heretics (or saints, for that matter) because of the way they smell. But we can take the bits of intuitive information the ancients gleaned and expand it under the light of modern science, because it is true that bad odors can make us sick and may even make us more prone to violence, which has an effect on our institutions. Hospitals, schools, and offices are all negatively affected when bad odors invade. For this reason, take care to avoid unpleasant odors in any learning environment you create.

Odors That Make Us Sick—Or Even Aggressive

In January of 1995, the Office of the Mayor of the city of Boston asked me to participate in a public hearing about a proposed site for an asphalt plant. On the face of it, this seems like an unremarkable event, yet the issues raised in this hearing are neither new to the world nor easily resolved. But nowadays, decisions about where to place commercial facilities that by their nature emit bad odors can—and should—be influenced by the knowledge we have gained about the effects of bad smells, or *malodors*, the word scientists use when discussing odors that may have a negative effect on large numbers of people.

In the case of the asphalt plant, we cited specific health concerns. For example, toxic odors can cause headaches, increase the incidence of asthma attacks, and adversely affect respiratory conditions. Unfortunately, ventures like paper mills, chemical plants, incinerators, and toxic waste sites are often placed in low-income neighborhoods, precisely where respiratory ailments such as asthma tend to be high in the first place. (As a result of community efforts, the location for the asphalt plant was not approved.)

We tend to think of exposure to noxious odors as an unusual event. But in the case of certain kinds of manufacturing and even farming, the bad smell may be present much of the time. What happens when an entire community is exposed to the same noxious smell, not on an occasional or accidental basis, but continually and deliberately? I once evaluated a town south of Chicago for the Attorney General's Office of the State of Illinois and the Illinois EPA (Environmental Protection Agency). It seemed that a mulching site for grass clippings had recently been located within the town, not far from a school. Depending on the way the wind blew, the horrible stench from the site blew toward the school and overwhelmed the children, not to mention the teachers. Naturally, a dispute arose over the odor and the location of the mulching site. Was the smell merely unpleasant, meaning that the people in the town could eventually adapt to it? Or was the bad odor so extreme that the school children's behavior was affected?

We found in our evaluation that teachers noted a far greater incidence of behavioral problems on the days that the wind blew the odor toward the school. This suggests that bad smells may indeed increase aggression, a theory supported by numerous other examples. Of course, aggression—and I'm using this word in the negative sense here—has many components. Until recently odors have been considered incidental and of little importance when we talk about violence. As we pull together information from numerous sources, however, we ignore the link between bad smells and aggression at our peril.

Destructive aggressive behavior always seems senseless, whether perpetrated by individuals or groups. Sometimes it seems inexplicable. For example, why would people enthusiastically attend a spectator sport, presumably for fun, but then engage in aggressive behavior that threatens the safety of everyone in the surrounding area? The extreme aggression on the part of some spectators during European soccer matches offers an example of the potential relationship between odors and aggressive behavior.

In the past, during the years when this soccer violence peaked, men comprised the vast majority of spectators and they stood while watching the game, usually drinking alcohol, too. They also tended to urinate where they stood. Because this behavior is so different from what generally takes place at other sporting events, it is logical to ask if the urine created such a bad smell over a period of time that it sparked fights between the male spectators. It is possible that bad odors directly act on the brain and become an important factor in inducing a violent emotional response.

The Odor Made Me Do It

In a now well-known study on aggression, Professor Robert Baron of Rensselaer Polytech Institute brought male college students into a room and told them that a contraption he devised was hooked up to a male "co-conspirator" in another room. By turning a knob on the contraption, the man in the other room would get an electric shock—and the perpetrator would hear a little scream. When no odor was introduced into the room, these students turned the knob to the right just a little bit, thereby keeping the level of electric shock to a minimum. But, when a bad smell was introduced to the room, they tended to turn the knob much farther, causing a more intense shock.

Some would say that all this shows is that male college students are suggestible and mean. But I believe this is one more piece of evidence demonstrating that we all are all susceptible to the influence of bad odors and may alter our behavior in the presence of a bad smell. For example, we know that on days when malodorous air pollution ratings are high, more automobile accidents are reported, suggesting that drivers are more aggressive and their usual caution is impaired in some significant way. In the era of "road rage," the odors inside your car may be important, too, especially if you tend to become irritable in heavy traffic. Keep the interior environment pleasant even if you have no control over traffic conditions.

The Warning Signs Are There

In order to measure the effects of bad odors on the brain, we undertook a study that measured brain waves coming from the limbic portion of the brain, which, as you recall, is also referred to as the emotional brain. We hooked up medical students to electroencephalogram (EEG) machines in order to measure brain waves and we used oxygen masks that were connected to an odorant through plastic tubing. When we introduced a very bad smell, galbanum, a smell similar to vomit, we documented a marked increase in amplitude of waves in the limbic portion of the brain and in the frontal lobes.

In this study, we did not attempt to measure how this change in brain waves affected behavior because we didn't want to induce aggression. We were simply trying to correlate a bad smell to changes in brain wave activity. However, when we performed a similar study on male athletes, we found that the presence of a bad smell increased the speed at which the men burned calories. We believe that the odor caused the athletes to become more stimulated, perhaps even aggressive, and led them to exercise with greater vigor. Who knows—perhaps one day we can constructively use the presence of a bad odor to harness or channel aggression to encourage more intense workouts, which would increase muscle strength and enhance the aerobic benefits. But while this might give new meaning to the phrase "no pain, no gain," most of us would not frequent a health club that floods its workout rooms with the odor of vomit. For the most part, we do not voluntarily hang out in malodorous places.

Our foundation is currently conducting a study involving professional and Olympic-class weightlifters. These athletes already sniff smelling salts just before a lift. Smelling salts give off the odor of ammonia, which irritates the trigeminal nerve and wakes people up. This is why smelling salts revive a person who has fainted, but most people would not choose to inhale that odor for pleasure. The purpose of our study is to determine if other odors will have the same effect as ammonia on the weightlifters. Perhaps a more pleasant odor will enhance performance, just as well as the less pleasant odor of ammonia.

Our work with the effects of unpleasant odors has taken us to prisons, schools, hog farms, paper mills, rubber plants, and to the sites of toxic chemical spills. Again and again, we have seen connections between how people behave, as well as the way they report feeling, based on their exposure to a bad smell.

Some combinations seem ripe for explosion. While we can't definitively say that bad odors will always make men, and perhaps women, more aggressive, why take unnecessary chances? When we evaluated a prison that was next to a garbage dump, we were looking at a situation where, on a statistical basis, a segment of our population already demonstrably prone to violence was being constantly exposed to a bad smell. Does this make sense in light of recent studies? I don't think so.

Fortunately, there were ways to correct the situation at the prison without moving either it or the dump. One could, for example, try to neutralize the smell of the dump, or alternatively, we could introduce pleasant odors into the prison. The French recently proposed putting the smell of flowers in their subways in an attempt to counteract the bad odor. Since most subway systems throughout the world smell less than pleasant, this seems like a worthy social experiment. Subways are common sites of crime, not solely because they smell bad, of course. They are also isolated and usually dark. However, introducing a pleasant smell to a subway system may turn out to be an inexpensive way to remove one of the factors that triggers aggression.

Getting rid of bad smells is a unique challenge in itself. Several years ago, the community of Buffalo Grove, Illinois, located north of Chicago, had a pig farm located across the street from a bank. The odor was extremely offensive and, naturally, the community wanted to remedy a situation that was threatening the bank's business. Fortunately, we came up with a solution that saved the pigs and the money. We added chlorophyll to the hog feed, thereby changing the smell of the pig's excrement. The odor was less strong and wasn't bothersome. All was fine, at least for a while, but the pig farm eventually closed and a used car lot took its place. (I leave you to decide who the winners and losers are in this story.)

As we learn more about the relationship between bad smells and aggression, we will have tools to make better choices about where we locate industrial plants, garbage dumps, stockyards, and the modern phenomenon of the factory farm. When we plan neighborhoods and communities, perhaps we will recognize that we promote aggressive behavior when we don't clean our streets and remove garbage from areas already stressed from poverty. And we may find ways to either neutralize the bad smells or introduce pleasant odors to make our environments more congenial and perhaps even less violent.

Can We Afford Bad Odors?

Since we are aware that bad odors have the potential to increase aggression and that bad odors are at the very least distracting and impair learning, we must think seriously about the odor atmosphere of certain kinds of environments. For example, psychiatric wards are notoriously malodorous. The windows are locked and the air becomes stale with the lingering scent of urine, and sometimes feces as well.

The patients on psychiatric wards are vulnerable to malodors because their ability to process incoming stimuli is distorted to begin with. When we work with psychiatric patients, we attempt to teach these men and women new ways of conceptualizing and processing human interactions. In an environment characterized by chronic bad odors, these individuals are less likely to have a successful psychotherapeutic experience. It is also likely that the unpleasant odors influence the hostile, aggressive behavior that occurs on psychiatric units.

We need to provide circumstances that *enhance* learning conditions in any environment meant to promote recovery and greater health, including nursing homes, which also tend to be permeated by bad odors. Other features of the environment may be designed to help the elderly retain cognitive skills and continue learning, but we need to give more attention to the "odor atmosphere." In addition, it stands to reason that malodors have a negative effect on staff, who may unconsciously equate smelling bad to being bad and respond to patients less positively when malodors dominate the environment.

Another instance in which a malodorous environment influences those who are already vulnerable takes place in our inner cities. This is particularly tragic because the children in this environment are already deprived of some valuable learning tools. To have their potential to learn further compromised by malodors disadvantages them even more. In addition, toxic waste facilities and incinerators are usually located in low-income areas because the residents often do not have the political clout to win battles to keep them out. These facilities add even more environmental stress to areas that are depressed economically and socially.

Malodors, Environmental Toxins, Health, and Memory

Chronic unpleasant odors, as well as chronic exposure to environmental toxins, have long-term consequences for health and for normal intellectual functioning. For example, it is known that chronic exposure to unpleasant odors from pulp mills can cause permanent olfactory loss. Bad odors can adversely influence mood, which over time can negatively affect the immune system. In addition, any strong odor can trigger an attack in individuals with unstable asthma. The negative effects of bad odors on mood state vary widely among individuals, and those who are already experiencing stress may be more vulnerable to unpleasant smells. What is mildly annoying to one person could even trigger aggressive behavior in a person already under stress.

There is a documented link between air quality and health status. In one study in which volunteers were exposed to unpleasant odors over time, these individuals experienced increased feelings of helplessness and their motivation to remedy the problem gradually diminished. In another study, women in Bavaria were asked to keep daily diaries describing their feelings of well being. The variations in how these women felt throughout the day coincided with changes in the quality of the air. Israeli researchers have also documented that health status is affected by air pollution. Furthermore, the longer people live in a polluted atmosphere, the less they notice it. Our ability to adapt is essential, but we may be adapting when it is not wise to do so.

The Consequences of Serious Environmental Toxins

Several years ago, the Smell & Taste Treatment and Research Foundation undertook a study of the effects of arsenic that was released into the air by a major industrial plant in College Station, Texas. The arsenic could be measured in dust on the ground and even in the houses. We performed extensive neurological testing on 169 individuals and found that the symptoms they showed were directly proportional to their distance from the plant, the length of time they lived in the area, and the level of arsenic on the ground near their homes. These individuals showed varying degrees of olfactory loss and decreased intellectual functioning and memory.

We initially began to suspect that there was significant neurological damage in these individuals because of what is known as the "reverse generational effect." In general, one sees better intellectual abilities and memory in the younger generations, which suggests that disease processes and aging have not affected mental capacities. However, in this situation, the reverse was true. The children, who were more likely to play in the dust and therefore had greater exposure to the arsenic at a vulnerable time of brain development, showed mental abilities that were not as good as those measured in adults. What this meant, of course, was that arsenic, an environmental toxin, was adversely affecting this community, most especially its growing children. Not all examples of environmental toxins are this extreme, but they alert us to the consequences of complacency and the results of ignoring the risks posed by some industrial sites.

Odors, Perceptions, and Attitudes

We know that people's perceptions of their environment are largely based on how it smells. We comment that a house smells clean or fresh. We say that we can't stay in a house another minute because of the bad pet odors. A table wax to which a lemon odor has been added is perceived more positively than one with no added smell. For the most part, this is a benign use of odors or preference.

A more malicious use of odor is evidenced by ascribing moral values to odors—which is learned behavior. We should not be too quick to judge our medieval ancestors as superstitious and ignorant. The sense of smell has been manipulated in more recent times. In general, it is relatively easy to convince people that something *is* bad because it *smells* bad. This can have serious consequences for societies. For example, our perceptions of homeless people may be distorted because they may not have the resources to meet the standard of cleanliness that we have developed over a long period of time in our society. Some people believe that a street person has less inherent worth as a human being, largely because he or she smells bad. From studies of the homeless, we know that most will go to extreme lengths to attempt to stay clean, precisely because they don't want to become even more isolated from mainstream life. But in the last 15 years or so, signs have appeared in public places stating: "Our restrooms are for customer use only," sending a message that homeless men and women are not welcome to clean up there. While this may be viewed as a necessary step on the part of business owners, in the long run it likely makes it more difficult for homeless people to pull themselves back up. In addition, the learned attitude about homeless individuals is perpetuated and today's children absorb it from their parents.

Some of today's street people are schizophrenics, who use

their bad smell to distance themselves from society or to keep us from intruding on their world. In this case, the person is using odor as a kind of primitive defense mechanism. We may not be able to do anything about the mentally ill person living in the park, but we may be more understanding of his or her situation when we grasp that the sense of smell may play a part in that person's perception of safety from others.

Many people cannot look beyond the odor of a person under any circumstances, even in themselves. If you believe you smell bad today—for whatever reason—you'll like yourself less than you do when you believe you smell good. Your self-esteem is affected by your perceptions of your breath, your body odor, and so forth. If you notice that an article of your clothing doesn't smell very good, your day is adversely affected and your perception of yourself may plunge.

Unfortunately, our rational capacities haven't completely eradicated the association between bad smells and bad people, or even evil people. One of the ugliest manifestations of this is when one group vilifies or isolates another group and uses odor as part of its excuse for hate.

In our own country, even in this century, African Americans were said to have a unique smell, giving the white power structure one additional justification for segregation, social ostracism, and even the Jim Crow laws that took so many years to eliminate. In the 1930s, Hitler said the same thing about the Jews. He claimed that they had a garlic-like smell, which when coupled with all the other vilifying claims, dehumanized them. The German propaganda machine also claimed that Gypsies had a bestial-like smell, and they too were one of Hitler's targeted groups. Once we allow the connection that we share a common humanity to weaken, the gate is opened for all manner of evil to take place.

What should give us pause is that manipulating and shaping these negative attitudes were shockingly easy. Populations were exposed to the information and failed to think it through; like other learned information, it influenced behavior. We need only look at human history to see that the sense of smell has played an important role in shaping prejudices.

Using the Knowledge We Have

Today, for the most part, bad odors present a health, behavior, and learning hazard that can be studied and remedied. As we amass more information, we can use it to plan our institutions and commercial ventures more wisely, and we can recognize that smells can, and often do, act on the brain and may contribute to ill health and also to the social problems we face. If we are wise, we will use our sense of smell to help us solve our difficulties rather than contributing to them.

Steps You Can Take

You can take some simple steps to prevent bad odors from interfering with learning and recall in your life:

+ *Control your learning environment by "sniffing out" bad odors. If you detect an unpleasant odor in your office or home, locate the source of it and remove it. Remember that your children are vulnerable to bad odors as well, so protect their studying environment, too.*

+ *Add pleasant odors to any learning situation—the floral odor is available to you now, but experiment with others, too.*

✦ *If you try to work or study during air travel, ask for seats as far away from the restrooms as possible. If you travel in first class, sit as far back in the cabin as possible; if you travel in coach, sit as far forward as you can, or, alternatively, near the exit row.*

✦ *Likewise, when you attend a large public gathering, avoid the portable restrooms as much as possible. Find a spot far away from those facilities.*

✦ *It may seem obvious, but pay attention to new industrial development in your community. Become involved in decisions about the placement of toxic waste sites and manufacturing plants that may affect air quality or emit unpleasant odors. Most certainly, pay attention to the location of schools relative to industrial or other potentially malodorous sites. Bad odors represent a community issue as well as an individual one.*

10

What Can Go Wrong?

Illness is the night-side of life,
a more onerous citzenship. Everyone who
is born holds dual citizenship, in the kingdom
of the well and in the kingdom of the sick.

— Susan Sontag

Unfortunately, some common diseases and conditions may lead to impairment of various types of mental functioning, including memory. So despite the fact that we can take steps to protect memory and mental capacities, some individuals will suffer from temporary or permanent loss of cognitive functioning.

Before I talk about what can go wrong, remember the fundamental principles that help you avoid—or at least delay—loss of mental abilities. You have control over many habits and behaviors that can cause memory impairment. A few of these activities include using illegal drugs, taking medications not specifically prescribed for you, excessive alcohol consumption, and smoking cigarettes. You can also take simple positive steps such as always using a seatbelt and wearing a bicycle or motorcycle helmet. Brain damage caused by head trauma (usually sustained in automobile accidents) may affect a variety of brain functions, including memory and the ability to learn and retain new information. Head trauma also is a common cause of damage to the olfactory nerves, sometimes leading to permanent loss of the ability to smell.

An additional step you can take is to engage in regular exercise. (Further discussion about the benefits of exercise appears in chapter 12.) You no doubt know that regular exercise promotes cardiovascular health and may help prevent hypertension (high blood pressure), diabetes, osteoporosis, and obesity. In fact, exercise is part of both treatment and prevention for these common diseases. Exercise serves as a "wild card" factor because it is associated with prevention and treatment of so many conditions. Recent research indicates that regular physical activity may even help prevent some of the devastating effects associated with the much-feared illness, Alzheimer's disease.

The Dreaded Disease

If we were to measure the "fear factor" involved in various illnesses, we would probably find that cancer and AIDS are the diseases most Americans of all ages fear most, but Alzheimer's disease (AD) likely comes in a close third. (The technical name of this illness is *senile dementia of the Alzheimer's type*.) Alzheimer's disease is devastating to the afflicted individual, as well as to family members and friends. About 25 percent of AD patients live in long-term care centers, and the remaining 75 percent are cared for at home.

Alzheimer's disease is the most common cause of dementia in the elderly population and, at any given time, it affects about 4 million individuals in the U.S. AD is responsible for about 75 percent of all cases of dementia among individuals 65 and older, and the risk for developing AD increases as we age. About 30 percent of men and women over age 85 develop AD. About 15 percent of affected individuals have a family history of the disease. Alzheimer's disease has been documented in childhood (among children with Down's syndrome), but 96 percent of cases occur in adults over age 40. (I know that sounds alarming, but the majority of cases occur in individuals over age 65.)

Perhaps what makes AD so dreaded is the fact that it is a progressive disease, with no known cure and little that can be done to stop the inevitable mental decline that usually takes place over a period of years. AD involves degeneration of brain neurons and a reduction in the size of the brain itself. Autopsies reveal abnormal tissue, or *senile plaques*, in the brain, as well as abnormal protein deposits, or *amyloids*, and the appearance of *neurofibrillary tangles*, a sign of degeneration of neurons.

AD progresses through four broad stages, although symptoms and rates of progression vary among individuals and stages may seem to overlap. The first stage is characterized by forgetfulness, and these early problems with memory often cause anxiety. An individual may begin making lists and find that more memory "systems" are required. Men and women find themselves posting reminder notes and keeping detailed calendars. Unfortunately, forgetfulness may lead to anxiety for individuals over age 40 or 50, who begin to associate every memory lapse as an indication of the onset of AD. However, the occasional memory lapse brought on by stress and the kind of work overload most people experience today should not be compared to the ongoing and increasing forgetfulness associated with developing Alzheimer's disease. Some change in social behavior may appear, and certain personality characteristics may intensify. A normally shy, quiet person, for example, may become noticeably withdrawn in social settings.

Patients and families gradually may realize something wrong in the first stage of the disease, but in the second stage memory loss becomes more severe and undeniable. Short-term memory is particularly affected; patients may remember the distant past, but be unable to recall an event that occurred earlier in the day.

Eventually, patients may become disoriented and restless, especially at night. Patients in this stage may pick at their clothes or fold and refold a handkerchief or scarf. Cognitive abilities decline in this stage and some individuals become unable to perform numerical calculations and may lack the ability to come up with even common words (dysphasia). AD patients may also experience a decrease in the ability to smell. Unfortunately, this stage is often marked by increasing anxiety and sometimes includes mood swings and personality changes.

The anxiety and depression we see among Alzheimer's patients may be related to the fact that the patients are aware of their declining abilities and quite naturally upset by them. To see one's mental capacities decline and realize personality changes are taking place may lead to understandable anxiety and depression.

During the third stage of AD, patients and families often experience great difficulties because the psychological symptoms usually worsen. Patients may suffer from hallucinations and delusions, which are symptoms of psychosis. Patients often receive care in institutions because personality changes can be severe in the third stage. At this point, AD patients may lack insight into their illness and also lose their sense of social norms. Unfortunately, some patients become unmanageable and even violent in this stage. In addition, physical decline often results in incontinence and patients no longer care about personal hygiene. Round-the-clock care is essential for patients in this stage of Alzheimer's disease.

The final stage of the disease is characterized by almost total unresponsiveness to caregivers, family members, and their surroundings in general. Some patients have volatile outbursts of laughing or crying, but eventually most AD patients withdraw and are out of touch with what we define as "the real world."

Many families have had some experience with Alzheimer's disease, including my own. My grandmother developed Alzheimer's while still in her sixties. I remember her telling hair-raising stories of her childhood prior to escaping from Russia and emigrating to the U.S. She could vividly recall— and recount—stories about hiding under her bed during the pogroms against the Jews in Russia. She had no recall, however, of what she had done the day before. Eventually, her declarative memory deteriorated, and she did not know the most basic general facts. Ultimately, even the episodic—autobiographical— memories vanished. Tragically, even procedural memory is subject to the devastation of Alzheimer's disease; my grandmother eventually forgot how to swallow and, hence, was unable to eat normally. She died in a nursing home, having long before lost the ability to recognize family members or even recall who she was. Such are the ravages of this disease.

The average lifespan from the time AD is diagnosed to death is about seven years, although 25 to 30 percent of AD patients live over 10 years. A smaller percentage live as long as 20 years. It is difficult to advise a family about the prognosis until the rate of progression has been observed over time.

What Causes Alzheimer's Disease?

To date we do not know the cause of AD. One theory about its origin postulates that a virus or toxin that invades the brain through the nose causes Alzheimer's. The olfactory pathway is one of the few areas in which the blood brain barrier does not exist. The blood brain barrier is a series of capillaries with tight junctions; their purpose is to prevent toxins, viruses, and bacteria from invading the brain. When we have an infection, even a common cold, it is rare that the infection invades the brain through the bloodstream.

The part of the brain that regulates nausea and vomiting is another area in which there is no blood brain barrier. This makes sense because a system designed to detect toxins early in the absorption phase of ingestion would need exposure to these toxins at high levels and as early as possible. The absence of a blood brain barrier allows these toxins to reach the brain faster and while still at low levels. The resulting nausea and vomiting empty the stomach before full absorption of the poison or toxin has occurred.

In addition, the pituitary gland, called the master gland, must be able to monitor or "sample" the levels of hormones in the body. For example, if more thyroid-stimulating hormone is needed, then the pituitary releases it directly into the blood. Thus, if the blood brain barrier existed here, the pituitary would not gain access to variations in hormone levels and then would not be an effective hormone "thermostat."

The theory linking the olfactory system to Alzheimer's disease postulates that whatever toxin causes the disease, it enters through the nose, at which point the toxin is absorbed in the mucosa and travels through the cribriform plate and enters the olfactory bulb. From there it affects the projections of the olfactory bulb, which means that the toxin then has a chance to "settle" in the hippocampi and the cortex, both of which control memory and mental functioning. This theory explains why and how AD damages the olfactory nerve and leads to the diminished ability to smell that is associated with the disease. The identity of the invading toxin remains in question, but aluminum silicate, found in sand, has been suggested as the culprit.

At one time, it was believed that the polio virus invaded the nose and spread to the brain. For this reason, some individuals began infusing zinc in the top of nose in order to destroy the olfactory nerve, thereby preventing the polio virus from entering.

This misguided use of zinc is not related to the fact that we need adequate zinc levels in the body to assure normal functioning of many systems of the body, including olfaction. In fact, zinc is a treatment for certain types of anosmia.

Recently, I have seen a cluster of patients who have lost their sense of smell through the use of an over-the-counter zinc inhaler, promoted as a way to prevent a cold. When zinc was discovered to act as a cold prevention measure, it was tested as an oral medication, not in the form of an inhaler. *If you use a zinc inhaler you run the risk of permanently losing your ability to smell. I recommend avoiding cold-prevention inhaling devices that contain zinc.*

Hope for a Cure

I wish I could report that a cure for Alzheimer's disease is on the horizon. Certainly, research continues for both effective treatments and preventive measures for this devastating disease. Currently, however, treatment tends to focus on controlling symptoms, monitoring nutritional status, and correcting deficiencies of certain B vitamins if necessary. To date, we use the few available drugs to slow the progression of the disease. Other medications, such as antidepressants and anti-anxiety drugs, are used to treat the psychological symptoms. As the disease progresses, it is important to control the Alzheimer's patient's environment to reduce confusion and simplify care as much as possible.

Within almost every community in our country, resources exist for patients and families of those suffering from Alzheimer's disease. Support groups have formed for family members and other loved ones. If your family is coping with Alzheimer's disease, I urge you to seek support and take advantage of community resources.

Other Causes of Dementia

The non-Alzheimer types of dementias share characteristics with AD, which makes diagnosis problematic in some cases. For example, symptoms of dementia, such as forgetfulness and changes in social behavior, may appear following strokes and develop as a result of heart disease, hypertension, and diabetes. In addition, many of the most common prescription and over-the-counter (OTC) drugs can induce confusion and impaired memory. It remains unclear if dementia is inevitable and perhaps even "normal" as we age. On one hand, some evidence suggests that if we live long enough we are likely to suffer some degree of dementia. A study conducted in the Netherlands reported that nearly everyone *over age 100* showed some evidence of cognitive decline. More than 70 percent of the "oldest old" had at least a moderate degree of dementia. Let's not forget, however, that 30 percent of men and women over age 100 do *not* show signs of dementia. Other studies have suggested that the prevalence of dementia among individuals age 95 and older is over 60 percent. Given that the current average lifespan is considerably less than 95 years for both sexes, dementia is avoidable for most people. (The Social Security Administration has projected that in the year 2050, life expectancy will be 82.9 years for women and 77.5 years for men. This represents a slight increase from 1995 figures of 79.0 for women and 72.6 for men.)

A variety of health problems contribute to decline in cognitive abilities. For example, in a 25-year study, men with hypertension experienced twice as much loss of intellectual functioning as did men with normal blood pressure. Athero-sclerosis and diabetes are also major causes of intellectual decline. We often associate hypertension and diabetes with strokes, but cognitive decline may occur in the presence of these conditions without the occurrence of stroke.

Avoiding a Stroke

Every year in the U.S., about 500,000 individuals experience a stroke, with effects ranging from mild to devastating. (Over 150,000 of these strokes are fatal.) Two major types of strokes exist: *ischemic* and *hemorraghic.* Ischemic strokes are the most common, accounting for 70 to 80 percent of the total number. These strokes occur when the blood supply to the brain is interrupted, whereas hemorraghic stroke occurs when a damaged vessel or artery ruptures in the brain. A stroke temporarily deprives selected brain cells of oxygen and glucose, causing them to die. Some strokes primarily affect physical functioning, and rehabilitation involves restoring or relearning basic skills such as walking or feeding oneself. In many cases, recovery is quite complete, but sometimes only partial recovery occurs.

Strokes that affect language and memory are obviously very serious. While some patients recover language skills (sometimes using melodic intonation therapy, discussed in chapter 3) and their ability to learn new information, other patients suffer permanent cognitive impairment. Obviously, prevention is key and the same factors that contribute to cardiovascular diseases and complications of diabetes put one at risk of stroke. High blood pressure is the most significant risk factor.

The Tragedy of Parkinson's Disease

About one in every 100 individuals in the United States will develop Parkinson's disease, which attacks a part of the brain called *substantia nigra.* The neurons in this region contain dopamine, a neurotransmitter involved in movement. Dopamine and acetylcholine are both necessary for normal bodily movement and, when functioning properly, the two neurochemicals maintain normal balance. In the presence of Parkinson's disease, however, the dopamine is deficient and muscles are unable to receive and process messages. Those with Parkinson's disease often experience an uncontrollable tremor, stiff movements, loss of balance, and eventually even the muscles in the face do not respond to ordinary "commands," such as smiling or even forming a frown.

Unfortunately, by the time the disease produces symptoms, the substantia nigra is almost completely destroyed. As with Alzheimer's disease, there is no cure for Parkinson's disease. Treatment includes taking drugs that inhibit acetylcholine or enhance dopamine. While these treatment approaches act to decrease symptoms, the disease process continues, so that eventually medications often yield little effect. In these situations, patients may be offered treatment with fetal cell implantation to the brain in order to enhance dopominergic nerve cells. This treatment has shown considerable success.

Other Disease States

A number of medical conditions negatively influence memory. For example, *Wernicke-Korsakoff's syndrome* results from severe malnutrition, specifically thiamine deficiency. It is a relatively rare but serious disease and for the most part occurs among individuals suffering from severe alcoholism. This disease has two parts, the first being Wernicke encephalopathy, which produces symptoms in many areas, including motor impairment, impaired reflexes, mental confusion, and abnormal eye movements. In the second stage, Korsakoff's psychosis, patients may suffer severe memory impairment, usually affecting recent memory but not necessarily distant memory. These patients may confabulate, meaning they invent stories that may be attempts to fill in the gaps in their memory. This is a serious disease and provides tragic evidence of severe consequences when alcoholism is left untreated.

The Faces of Amnesia

The notion of amnesia has fed the imagination of many novelists and film producers. The idea that we can experience a traumatic event, such as a head injury, and lose all memory of the past, even our personal history, has the power to intrigue as well as frighten. In actuality, complete loss of memory is quite rare, but transient forms of amnesia can occur under a variety of conditions.

Seizures are abnormal electrical activities in the brain, and a number of medical conditions can cause them. Most people associate seizures with epilepsy, but strokes and head injuries can cause seizure activity, too. Not all seizures affect memory, but those that occur in the temporal lobe will cause amnesic state or difficulty with immediate recall. Seizure activity may interfere with memory because of impaired hippocampal function. During these episodes, patients may be confused and unable to process new information, and a form of amnesia occurs.

With *retrograde amnesia,* the individual has no memory of the episode itself and sometimes of what happened even before the event. With *antegrade amnesia,* no memory exists about what happened after the trauma. However, memory can return after a period of time. In chapter 2, I described being hit by a car while riding a bicycle when I was a medical student. Immediately after the accident, the last thing I recalled was being at the top of the hill, but I was hit at the bottom of the hill. I also had antegrade amnesia for the period after being hit and before the ambulance arrived. Years later, I recalled the car coming toward me, but the last 15 seconds or so before impact have never come back to me. So, I still have retrograde amnesia for a small portion of the episode.

Short-term amnesia manifests in a variety of ways. I was once called to appear on the *Jerry Springer Show* and participate as an expert on memory. One of the guests had no short-term memory at all, a situation that resulted from destruction of both hippocampi. This guest had to write down the name of every person she met, and without her notebook she would have no memory of having met the person just a few minutes earlier. Her long-term memory remained intact, but she was unable to learn any new information.

The second guest on that program suffered from *psychogenic amnesia*. She had hit her head, lost her memory, and years later she found herself living in a different city. She had married and had a different family and was unaware of her situation until she was hit on the head again and memories of her other life returned and she realized she had two families. I call this type of situation the "Gilligan's Island syndrome," because it is reminiscent of an episode in that television series. A coconut falls on Gilligan and he loses all memory of himself and his fellow castaways. In this condition, he winds up foiling an attempted rescue of his shipwrecked friends. The episode ends when another coconut falls on his head and he again remembers his stranded friends from the *SS Minnow*. This type of amnesia can be treated with psychotherapy or amytal (truth serum).

Amnesia can be an organic problem rather than one of psychiatric origin. I once treated a patient who reported spells of amnesia lasting 15 to 25 minutes. During these episodes, he felt anxious, but continued to walk around, sometimes asking inappropriate questions, although he was never combative with those around him. This patient described himself as confused, and before the incidents occurred he experienced the phenomenon of déjà vu, a situation in which individuals feel as if they have lived the current incident before. He could sometimes link the onset of an episode with having a cocktail or eating a big meal. They also occasionally happened after exercise or if he stayed up especially late. Between these attacks, he had no memory impairment. Extensive testing (glucose tolerance testing, Magnetic Resonance Imaging [MRI], neuropsychiatric tests, psychological tests, and blood and urine studies) led to a diagnosis of transient global amnesia, or retrograde amnesia. This patient was able to cope once he understood what was happening to him. Fortunately, this type of transient amnesia is relatively uncommon.

Consciousness, Smell, and Memory

During deep sleep we recall fewer dreams than during light sleep. For the most part, your sense of smell sleeps along with you. However, an odor can awaken you, if the smell has a component to stimulate the trigeminal nerve, such as the odor of ethyl mercaptin, the chemical that is added to natural gas to give it a detectable smell. The odor of ammonia in smelling salts also rouses you by stimulating the trigeminal nerve.

Level of consciousness affects your ability to remember. Catatonia is a state in which a person is awake, yet totally unresponsive to the outside world. The first catatonic patient I took care of was in this unresponsive state for many months. I saw her many times and talked to her, but she showed no response at all. After she had electroshock therapy, she "woke up" and was able to describe to me what she recalled during all our sessions.

An intriguing area of memory and consciousness involves the ability to recall information even in a state of very low consciousness. After regaining consciousness, coma patients may recall the music family members played for them. During gallbladder surgery, patients under anesthesia and wearing earphones could not hear what the surgeon and others were saying in the operating room; these individuals recovered faster than those who did not wear the earphones. These cases, and others like them, show that the brain is capable of recording information even when we do not make a choice to pay attention.

Ganser's Syndrome

Ganser's syndrome is a special case. In essence, it is the intentional distortion of mental functioning. In other words, situations exist in which individuals intentionally make mistakes in memory recall and cognition. These individuals have an ulterior motive, such as getting out of the draft, avoiding a prison term, or extending worker compensation claims. When describing what they did a year before, they will come up with answers that are approximations of the truth, almost complete or correct. Their behavior is supposed to look like an organic dysfunction, but it is essentially a faked "disorder." Individuals who engage in this behavior are known as *malingerers*, and usually the motivation is simple self-interest. Fortunately, we have a variety of tests that "catch" malingerers. These tests include neurological tests, including "scratch 'n sniff" smell testing, and other physical examinations and written tests.

Most of the time malingering serves no positive purpose, and when all is said and done, it represents just another form of dishonesty. However, I was involved in a case in which a man engaged in malingering for what turned out to be an excellent reason. I was called in to examine a death row inmate, whose execution by lethal injection was schedule for only two days away. His defense team had claimed his I.Q. was very low and the Illinois Supreme Court ordered testing to establish his mental competency.

Within a few hours, I could clearly see he was malingering. During the formal verbal tests, he was barely responsive, but he was known to talk to other inmates on death row and play chess regularly. Meanwhile, some students from a local university, who had been working nonstop on this case, finally obtained a videotaped confession from the actual murderer and my "patient" was set free—literally within hours of his execution.

As a result of this case, and it was indeed a close call, Governor James Ryan issued an executive order that put a moratorium on all executions in Illinois. This case made national news, but I do not believe most people were aware that the innocent man engaged in malingering behavior, which in his case involved pretending to be mentally incompetent in order to delay his execution until the students could hunt down the real murderer. I guess one could say that malingering has its uses!

The Special Case of Depression

Depression deserves special attention. First, it is a very common psychiatric illness and it negatively influences all phases of learning and memory, including the ability to concentrate. Equally important, depression can creep up, so to speak, and many individuals do not realize they are depressed. In a sense, they adapt to functioning at a lower level and eventually it feels normal. Of course, reduced energy and occasional sleep disturbances do not necessarily mean that depression is present. Likewise, life events can sometimes cause sadness and lack of concentration. An occasional symptom does not point to depression; it's the persistence of a symptom that may indicate depression. I devised this self-test as a *screening test only*. If your answers point to a *possible* hidden, underlying depression, I suggest you see your personal physician for a complete evaluation.

1. Are you in a sad or depressed mood most of the day?

2. Do you feel sad or empty?

3. Are you less interested in things in your life, including the activities you used to find pleasurable?

4. In the last month, have you lost more than five percent of your body weight without trying to?

5. Has your appetite changed? Do you either want to eat more or less than normal every day?

6. Do you have trouble sleeping well?

7. Do you sleep excessively and have trouble getting up and starting your day?

8. Do have a feeling of restlessness?

9. Do you feel fatigued?

10. Is your energy level consistently low?

11. Do you feel worthless?

12. Do you feel guilty almost all the time?

13. Are you increasingly indecisive?

14. Do you have trouble concentrating?

15. Do you have recurrent thoughts of death?

16. Do you ever feel like hurting yourself?

Answering "yes" to any of these questions could point to depression, and I recommend that you consult with your physician to discuss this potential difficulty.

The Brain Is Resilient

Despite the potential for serious memory loss and disorders that prevent learning and retention, the brain is actually incredibly resilient and adaptable. Damage to one area does not necessarily result in total loss of function because another part of the brain assumes the function of the damaged area. In other words, the brain can redirect and relearn abilities. Several years ago, I had a patient named Luanne, whose parents brought her in for an evaluation because of her severe headaches and also because she stumbled more than is normally expected in childhood. When I evaluated her, I observed a wide gait and that she could not walk a straight line. Magnetic resonance imaging (MRI) revealed a large tumor in the cerebellum, the region of the brain that controls motor function and in which our motor skill memories are stored. Luanne's cerebellum was almost completely replaced by the tumor. After undergoing surgery that removed both the tumor and her cerebellum, she still did not function normally. However, months and years after the surgery her motor ability became very close to normal. After five years, she is able to walk, run, and ride a bicycle without difficulty.

With the exception of injuries, most people do not give much thought to brain function or to the capacity to learn and retain new information. Most of us take our mental abilities for granted. This begins to change as we grow older, a time when any sign of decline begins to trigger uneasy feelings, perhaps even fear of losing mental capacities. In the next chapter, I will talk about normal aging processes and offer suggestions about the best way to stay mentally fit throughout your life.

11

Memory, Learning, and Normal Aging

The man who thinks over his experiences most and weaves them into systematic relations with each other will be the one with the best memory.

— William James

Most of us know elderly individuals whom we describe as remarkable. These men and women seem to defy the stereotypes about aging and we tend to both admire them and hope to emulate the way they have coped with growing older. For me, the person who will always stand out is Elizabeth Crosby, one of my professors in medical school at the University of Michigan. She was 99 when I took her neuroanatomy course, and she was 102 when she wrote her last textbook. She was a highly respected professor and apparently the word "retirement" was not in her vocabulary. Of course, Dr. Crosby sounds remarkable, but she was actually normal. The image of older people languishing in nursing homes, unable to recognize family members or suffering with serious memory loss, is not an image of *normal* aging. Rather, it is a picture of pathology— illness. Our challenge as we grow older is to do everything we can to maintain normal function and avoid pathology.

In 2002, the American Association of Retired Persons (AARP) celebrated their 44th anniversary. The AARP has made our society more conscious than ever before of the needs of older people in our society. With 77 million baby boomers in their forties and fifties, we see increasing attention focused on changing lifestyles among the older population. In a poll of baby boomers, the AARP reports that eight of ten men and women said they intend to work at least part-time after age 65. Some plan to work because they expect to need the income; others intend to start businesses; still others want to continue working because they enjoy it. Currently, only 12 percent of people over age 65 are in the work force, so over the next two decades, the face of the workplace across the United States is going to take on a different look.

Even before the AARP survey, expectations about aging clearly are undergoing great changes. Developing a more positive attitude about growing older and our increasing recognition that aging by itself does not automatically lead to a profound loss of mental or physical abilities represent beneficial trends in our society. However, active, healthy older years are not guaranteed, nor should longevity be a goal in itself. In order to live fully as you age, whatever your ultimate lifespan turns out to be, you must begin now to prevent diseases and conditions that threaten to rob you of your vitality—and, in some cases, rob you of a sharp memory.

Put Your Fear in the Right Place

Most people worry about developing Alzheimer's disease in their later years. Indeed, this is one of the biggest fears among the middle-aged as well as the elderly. Along with the dreaded Alzheimer's disease, most people in their middle years begin to imagine mental and physical deterioration that could lead to loss of independence and eventual confinement in a care center for the aged. When asked, most people say they would like to live an active life until they quietly die in their sleep—preferably before major deterioration sets in. The biggest fears are (1) losing one's ability to think clearly and retain information previously learned and (2) diminished ability to acquire new information.

It appears that most people expect to face some memory loss and even reduced cognitive dysfunction as they age. Somerset Maugham is said to have opened a lecture by stating that there were many positive things about aging, and after a long pause he said, "I'm just trying to think what they are." There is a natural human tendency to try to laugh instead of cry, so to speak, when facing something that has great emotional impact—even our greatest fear.

Unfortunately, many people believe that loss of intellectual functioning is inevitable and, once experienced, is irreversible. However, this is not the case, which is the reason I direct this chapter to readers of all ages. It has been well established that how you live today will influence the quality of your life tomorrow. For people who envision new careers and part-time jobs and perhaps meaningful volunteer work and travel in their later years, it is never too early or too late to focus on prevention. Of course, overcoming stereotypes about aging is important too.

Expectation versus Reality

Samuel Johnson once pointed out that if a young person forgets a name or a common fact, no one thinks much about it, but if an older person forgets the same things, people immediately begin to feel pity because it's clear that the person's "memory is going." The older person may think that this kind of memory lapse is a big deal too.

An interesting study demonstrated that, in our culture, the expectation of "failing" memory could lead to the reality. Becca Levy and Ellen Langer, both from Harvard University, compared memory function in a group of older deaf people with that of elderly subjects with normal hearing. Presumably, the deaf individuals were not as likely to have been as deluged with negative stereotypes about aging, whereas those with normal hearing would have been more profoundly influenced by our culture's expectations of memory loss. And, as it turned out, Levy and Langer's hypothesis was correct. The deaf Americans had better memories than those with normal auditory function. Levy and Langer also compared memory function of older American subjects with elderly Chinese citizens, whose culture generally shows greater respect for the elderly and for aging itself. This group performed better than older Americans and their memories were shown to be as good as young Chinese men and women who were also tested—and hearing-impaired older Americans.

The implication is that the assumption in our culture that older people will experience increased forgetfulness leads to greater memory loss, and also to more concern about it. Samuel Johnson was correct to point out that a memory lapse in older age is in our culture considered a noteworthy "event." Recently, we have begun to hear the term "senior moment" to describe an episode in which a particular word or name just won't appear at will.

While it is true that there is a "benign forgetfulness of senescence," or normal memory loss with aging, that can be demonstrated and measured, most of us have exaggerated fears of loss of cognitive functioning. Certain brain disorders will result in decreased mental functioning regardless of age, but a relatively small percentage of us will fall victim to these disorders. And, as discussed in the previous chapter, head trauma at any age can lead to impaired intellectual functioning. However, there is a vast difference between age-associated dementia or Alzheimer's disease and the normal forgetfulness associated with growing older. About 25 percent of men and women over the age of 80 suffer from some form and degree of dementia. Looked at another way, 75 percent of this population do not suffer from any form of dementia. In one study, approximately 60 percent of elderly people met criteria for age-associated memory impairment. (The mean age was 72.) However, only 9 percent of those with age-associated memory impairment developed any form of dementia, including Alzheimer's disease.

Forgetting a word now and then or having difficulty recalling some previously known fact is a far cry from the pathologic state of age-associated dementia or senile dementia of the Alzheimer's type. Furthermore, you can do many things to prevent memory loss and a decrease in intellectual functioning as you age.

Expectations of aging may unconsciously influence our behavior and mental capacities. You may have heard older individuals, and sometimes even middle-aged men and women say things like: I'm too old to dance, take a class, surf the Web, change careers, learn a language, change my attitudes, and so forth. If we believe we're too old to change our lifestyle or adopt new attitudes or learn new skills, then in a sense we probably are. However, research suggests that if we regularly exercise the brain, then functioning can actually improve.

Several years ago, in a study conducted at Harvard University, men ages 75–80 were taken to a rural retreat for a five-day experiment. These men were divided into two groups, with the first group instructed to pretend that it was 1959. The men were told to act, talk, and think the way they did in 1959, and radio and television programs were provided to help them travel back to the atmosphere of that time. They even watched the movie *Anatomy of a Murder* and listened to the voice of President Eisenhower on a taped speech. Participants in the other group were instructed just to talk and reminisce about their lives back in 1959.

The men who spent five days acting as if they were actually living in 1959 showed improvement on intelligence test scores and on tests that measured reaction time. The group that only talked about that year either remained the same or showed some decline. This study suggests that living as a younger person, even for a short time, can alter mental functioning for the better. So it is possible that with concentrated effort some cognitive decline may be reversible, and achieving some improvement may not take months or years. A group of men and women ages 64–95 showed significant improvement in mental functioning after undergoing just five one-hour sessions that focused on abstract reasoning and mental speed.

Prevention Is the Key

Rather than listing all the possible diseases and disorders you could develop as you age, thereby increasing your concern, I prefer to look at the optimistic side of the picture. As a result of longitudinal studies, we can assemble a list of positive factors that increase the chances for sharp mental functioning as we age. We may not have control over our genes, but we do have control over many of the elements that increase our chances for vigorous and healthy aging—and a sharp memory. Each factor listed below is important, and I recommend using them as guidelines to assess your life and your lifestyle.

Take steps to prevent chronic diseases, including cardiovascular disease

Given what is known about preventing diseases of the cardiovascular system, there is no excuse for not adopting a heart-protective lifestyle. While a full discussion of this is outside the scope of this book, barely a day goes by without new evidence that a diet low in saturated fat can lower cholesterol or keep cholesterol levels low, which in turn can lower the risk of developing heart disease.

In addition, cigarette smoking is one of the primary risk factors for not only cardiovascular disease, but also for lung, throat, and oral cancers and a host of other problems, including emphysema. Cigarette smoking also decreases the amount of oxygen delivered to the brain. If you are a smoker and need further motivation to quit, consider that *smoking increases your chances of heart disease and decreased intellectual functioning down the road.*

Ideally, a heart-protective lifestyle should begin in childhood, but it is never too late to begin changing destructive lifestyle habits and discussing heart disease prevention strategies with your physician. While a low total cholesterol level (preferably under 200) is not an absolute guarantee that you will not develop heart disease, it is a sensible goal and a place to begin. (Unfortunately, there are no definitive studies about the effects of high cholesterol on men and women over age 70, so no one can yet say what the optimal level is in older people.) Stay away from all tobacco products—including those trendy cigars that some men, and even a small percentage of women, have begun to brandish. Women as well as men should be concerned about heart disease; cardiovascular disease is a "killer" disease for both sexes.

A heart-protective lifestyle also includes regular exercising and avoiding recreational drugs such as cocaine. It is generally accepted that very moderate alcohol intake (one drink per day or so) may be beneficial to the heart, but I am not recommending that anyone who currently does not use alcohol begin drinking. We know that excessive alcohol use increases the risk of heart and liver diseases as well as contributes to memory loss and decreased intellectual functioning. Alcohol intake is also linked with increased risk of breast cancer, and olfactory acuity also decreases as alcohol intake increases.

Chronic, long-term use of alcohol is known to produce olfactory loss, but the immediate effect has not been measured until recently. We undertook an unusual study with four volunteers, employees of the State of Illinois, to measure the relationship between inebriation and olfaction. In other words, we asked these volunteers to get drunk and we measured their ability to smell before their first drink and in between drinks. We also gave them cognitive tests. In addition, state troopers administered Breath Alcohol Analyzer tests to measure blood alcohol levels. Our volunteers were free to pick their favorite drink; one chose tequila and lime juice, one chose rum pina coladas, the third chose rum daiquiris, and the fourth chose beer. Each drink contained the equivalent of 0.8 ounces of pure alcohol. As our testing progressed, all showed signs of inebriation and the more they drank, the worse their sense of smell became. Three of the four individuals drank enough (four double drinks for the tequila and daiquiri drinkers and 6.5 beers for the fourth person) to reach the legal limit for driving, which in Illinois was 0.10 percent blood alcohol content. Our pina colada drinker never reached that because she passed out when her level was 0.095. We don't know why the sense of smell progressively diminishes as alcohol consumption increases, but alcohol may act as a toxin to the olfactory system, similar to other toxins such as lead, hydrogen sulfide, and arsenic.

Encouraging public employees to get drunk may seem like a frivolous endeavor, but our study has practical implications. For example, since 90 percent of taste is smell, if you drink alcohol before preparing or eating a meal, you may miss the subtle aromas and flavors of foods. Most of the snacks served in bars tend to be salty, probably because patrons can taste the salty pretzels and peanuts and chips after their ability to taste most foods has diminished. Many older people complain that food begins to taste bland as they age, and this occurs because of diminished olfactory ability. Since your sense of smell diminishes with age, you may want to curtail alcohol before a meal or even with a meal in order to retain full enjoyment of your meals.

Stay mentally stimulated and active

One of the most important messages of this book is that stimulating the brain keeps it fine-tuned and humming along throughout life. As I've said before, watch television less and read more. Play word games—don't throw away the Scrabble board. Test your memory by watching *Jeopardy* and invite your friends and neighbors in for a game of Trivial Pursuit.

I realize that many men and women do stay active in their later years, and I do not mean to insult individuals for whom the term "slowing down" is meaningless. Many people in our society already have taken the late George Burns's advice and have chosen not to retire. Millions of older adults use their later years to develop new interests, begin or expand volunteer activities, or learn new skills. However, since our society tends to encourage passivity and inactive lifestyles in people of all ages, everyone can use a reminder to choose active physical and mental pursuits.

Use some the tips and activities in this book to help you stay active. Learn something new by using "In Just 15 Minutes a Day," or start the "7-Minute Workout." Keep a journal or start writing your life story. (See "Leave a Written Legacy" on page 231.) Use the odorized bookmark when you work on mentally challenging projects. For the most part, you do not need to create artificial activities to stay sharp. Most of us can find plenty of mental stimulation by reading, listening to music, learning or continuing to play an instrument, learning a new skill, managing our finances, traveling, or taking classes at adult learning centers. Some seniors find travel a mentally stimulating activity, particularly if it is travel with a purpose, such as educational tours offered through organizations such as Elderhostel.

High socioeconomic status—a favorable environment

In general, we have limited control over this, and it is also a relative concept. Most of us are not and never will be fabulously wealthy celebrities or CEOs whose incomes boggle the mind. But, as a group, the large middle class in the United States usually has sufficient economic resources to maintain flexibility about where and how they live. This group also has access to basic health care as well as educational and recreational services. One needn't be wealthy to exercise, stimulate the mind, or live in a relatively comfortable environment. It is true that the very poor in our society have less control over basic environmental factors and these individuals may have more limited choices. Recent research has confirmed that just being poor in our culture is a significant factor in premature death. Any other lifestyle issues, such as diet and exercise, are not as statistically significant as low economic status.

One way to look at health and socioeconomic status is to look at *individuals.* We all know rich people who died young and alone and poor people who celebrated their 100th birthday surrounded by loving family. We think about our own health, not in the context of a group, but as a personal issue. We tend to calculate our personal risk factors and evaluate the results of our medical tests. Your family physician views you as an individual, too. However, when we take a societal view of health, we face puzzling issues. An essay for the "My Turn" column in N*ewsweek* magazine by Stephen Bezruchka, MD, published in February 2001, raised questions that apply to our society as a whole, taking us out of the realm of looking at health on an individual basis.

As you probably know, countries are ranked according to various statistics, such as infant mortality and life expectancy. In 1970 the U.S. ranked twentieth in the world, but by 1990 we had dropped to twenty-fifth. Dr. Bezruchka views the widening gap between rich and poor as at least partially responsible for this drop. Japan, on the other hand, has enjoyed steadily rising life expectancy and currently ranks *number one*. In the years after World War II, Japan not only enjoyed great economic expansion, but it also structured the economy to allow all its citizens to share more equally. As the gap between the rich and poor narrowed, life expectancy increased. It has always seemed puzzling that smoking, for example, has decreased in the U.S., and twice as many Japanese men as American men smoke—yet the U.S. has *twice* as many deaths attributable to smoking. It has become increasingly clear that we can institute various "life-saving" health measures and continue to develop sophisticated medical technology unknown in much of the world, but we are not likely to appreciably change our longevity statistics without reconsidering our widening gap between rich and poor.

Have a flexible personality in middle age

One's basic personality is difficult to change, but we can stay mindful of our strengths and weaknesses and expand our personality. Perhaps the best way to look at this is to avoid staying in the proverbial "rut." Boredom and rigidity tend to lead to decreased mental sharpness; change and being open to new ideas stimulate the brain. Older people who are learning to use computers and can teach the rest of us about the wonders of the World Wide Web are obviously people who remain open to new ideas.

Take steps to maintain vision and hearing

This is as simple as having regular eye exams and screening to detect gradual hearing loss. Just think of the superior hearing aids available today and the rapid advances in cataract surgery, for example. Is there any excuse not to avail yourself of the latest medical and technological advances that can help keep these senses sharp?

Maintain a high level of perceptual processing speed

Perceptual processing speed is what is required to be a champion video game player—among other things. This skill does tend to diminish with age, so my advice is to spend a few minutes now and then playing video games with your grandchildren or visit the game room in the local mall and ask some teenagers to show you around. Maybe one day, we will see game rooms specifically designed for older people!

Learn to be satisfied with your accomplishments in life

If this sounds easier said than done, bear in mind that there was only one Mother Teresa. Most of us do our life's work without notoriety and if we compare ourselves to others, we might wonder if our life has mattered. For most people, long-term life satisfaction comes from raising children; maintaining friendships; knowing they did their job well, whatever it was; or through helping a few people when they could. Living with great regret or feeling cheated and negative about how we've lived tends to take much away from one's later years.

Younger people should periodically assess their lives and attempt to change the things that can be changed. If a job is making you miserable, either change your attitude toward it or find another job. If relationships are strained, attempt to repair them. If you know you have undeveloped abilities or talents, do what you can to nurture these untapped attributes. Carrying a bundle of regrets into your later years may be detrimental to your health.

In recent years, community colleges, universities, and other learning centers have started various courses in "conscious aging." That term generally encompasses an attitude that accepts the reality of growing older and resisting the tendency to "worship" youth. This does not mean embracing a downhill slide—far from it. Rather, these classes often help men and women find their new and vital role in their families and societies. The emphasis on conscious aging recognizes that older people have much to offer the generations behind them, but the ability to redefine one's important role in a new phase of life often depends on a willingness to come to terms with the past. If you find yourself at a crossroads in late midlife, I suggest taking one of these classes in order to explore a new vision and new goals for your later years.

Be married to a person who functions at a high intellectual level

Well, this last item may be advantageous but I certainly don't recommend divorcing one partner and looking for another who is more intellectually stimulating! In general, we know that warm, positive relationships are important in maintaining good health. The support of a compatible and loving spouse, who also functions well intellectually, is great if you have it. If you happen to be married to a person who is not interested in sharpening his or her mind, then choose activities that you enjoy and pursue them on your own. And single people can form friendships or increase their contact with loved ones and reap benefits, too. Single or married, the most important thing is to stay involved with other people and engage in a wide range of activities.

For a Sharp Mind, Move Your Body

Exercise is so important that it merits additional attention. Ideally, exercise programs should begin early in life and be maintained through one's older years. On a hiking trip in Tuscany, I met the Cowens, a couple (one is 60, the other 80) who walk five miles a day, every day, unless the snow is so deep it blocks their front door. The only "symptom" of aging they experience is what they call a "gradual slowing down." (Up into their 70s, they took hiking vacations in which they covered up to 15 miles a day.) Neither partner takes any medication for any disorder. I consider them role models for us all.

The benefits of exercise extend beyond anecdotal reports. In one study, participants in a walking program for only 26 days performed better on memory tests than those in the control group, comprised of individuals who did not exercise regularly. Another study documented the relationship between physical activity and stroke prevention. The protective effect of exercise against stroke was found in both men and women, younger and older people, and in all racial and ethnic groups. A Finnish study of approximately 16,000 men and women, age 25–64, showed a positive effect of exercise in a lowered death rate, even after taking other lifestyle and genetic factors into consideration.

What all these studies suggest is that physical activity is critical to long-term health and has implications for retaining mental acuity. At any age, individuals who are physically fit and active perform better on tests of cognitive function. If you are in your twenties, thirties, or forties and have let yourself become a couch potato, it is time to change your ways. The Centers for Disease Control and Prevention and the National Institutes of Health recommend thirty minutes of moderately intense physical activity per day. Brisk walking—brisk enough to elevate the heart rate—is probably the most accessible exercise for everyone.

No good excuses exist to avoid starting an exercise program. Some shopping malls open their doors early in the morning to accommodate fitness walkers, and video stores carry exercise tapes suitable for all ages and fitness levels. Many people have exercise bicycles in their homes, but they are using them as clothing racks or hiding them away in the basement. It's time to dust off the exercise equipment or just start walking. If you are out of shape and haven't exercised in a long time, start by walking ten minutes a day and gradually increase to thirty minutes. Most people can increase their walking time to an hour. Swimming is not considered a fat-burning exercise, but it is beneficial in that it does not put strain on joints and bones. For this reason, elderly individuals often prefer it.

Exercise programs such as yoga and tai chi increase flexibility and help keep the body supple and graceful. These exercises also promote relaxation and increase the ability to focus and concentrate. Many senior centers and health clubs offer these gentle forms of exercise in classes designed for older people. Ideally, you should begin them when you are still young and have full range of motion in your joints and muscles, but don't let age stop you from increasing your fitness level. (Of course, check with your physician before you start any exercise program.)

Two benefits of exercise have a direct link to memory and intellectual functioning. Exercise promotes increased oxygen levels in the brain, which in turn is associated with improved mental functioning. Second, exercise directly stimulates the central nervous system, meaning that the mechanisms that control mental capacities are stimulated.

Obesity and Inactivity

Perhaps what should alarm us all is the relative inactivity among children. Both childhood and adult obesity are on the rise. Nowadays, children rarely engage in vigorous exercise except if they play an organized sport. Just a few decades ago, I routinely walked or cycled three miles to attend school; today, I drive my children to school or they are picked up by a school bus. It is rare to see young people using bicycles as a primary means of transportation. These changes would not be detrimental if other activities were taking their place, but this is not happening. Too many children spend most of their free time in front of television, not playing outside on the street with friends or in their backyards. Shari, a neighbor, commented about how rare it is to see children playing on the sidewalk in our neighborhood. I do not think we can blame the children for this trend toward sedentary lifestyles. We are the adults, the role models, and we need to look at our own habits before we shake our heads and conclude that today's children are just lazy!

Obesity is associated with high blood pressure, increased risk for stroke and cardiovascular (heart) diseases, and higher incidence of adult onset diabetes. Conversely, normal weight is associated with lower incidence of all these conditions. Looking at the collective data, one can only conclude that exercise plays a major role in achieving and maintaining normal weight and preventing or delaying the onset of the degenerative diseases that have for too long been considered "normal" diseases of aging. Unfortunately, these same diseases are implicated in decline in mental function. In actuality, if we prevent or delay these conditions and illnesses, we have made a huge stride in preserving memory and high intellectual functioning.

Blood Pressure and Memory

According the National Institute on Aging, middle-aged individuals with high blood pressure are more likely to have problems with their memory as they age. For this reason, it is important to have your blood pressure checked regularly, and if you have high blood pressure take immediate steps to lower it. As you probably know, elevated blood pressure (hypertension) is associated with increased risk of stroke and heart disease. Less widely known is that persistent hypertension can impair intellectual functioning among the elderly.

One longitudinal study tracked 3,735 men over thirty years. The average age of the participants was 48 at the beginning and 78 at the end of the study. Men who had high systolic blood pressure (the higher of the two numbers in a blood pressure reading) in middle age were 2.5 times more likely to have difficulties with memory and other intellectual functions than were men with normal blood pressure. In some cases, diet, exercise, quitting smoking, and stress management can lower blood pressure. However, medication may be necessary to treat hypertension in many cases. This is not an area to ignore or leave to chance. Self-care programs, including a regular exercise program and reduced sodium in the diet, are necessary even if medication is required.

The odor of green apple, which has been studied for its ability to reduce anxiety and prevent or alleviate migraine headaches, also tends to lower blood pressure. While it is not available as a treatment yet, I believe that within this decade the beneficial effects of certain odors will be so well documented that some will be used therapeutically and the age of true aromatherapy will be upon us.

Change in Cognitive Functioning Varies

In popular literature, changes in cognitive functioning tend to be described as if mental abilities were one entity. This implies that mental sharpness in all areas declines at about the same rate. However, it is important to note that some mental abilities improve after young adulthood and, in general, overall intellectual competence peaks in the forties and fifties; in some mental skills, the subsequent decline is slow and uneven. For example, verbal abilities tend to increase with age and change very little in early old age. Although numeric ability tends to decrease with age, the average older American outperforms today's high school graduates because they developed greater numerical skills in school and beyond.

Apparently, numeric ability reached a peak level among individuals born around 1917 and there has been a gradual decline ever since. (It is not your imagination that many of today's young people do not know how to make change at a cash register. The computerized registers perform this task, but when the technological glitch inevitably occurs, the back-up skill is notably absent.) Numeric skills are also among those less exercised today because we have pocket calculators. We are training future generations to be numerically impaired. As part of my daughter Marissa's second-grade math homework, she was given simple addition tabulation problems and was told to use a calculator to solve them.

The slide rule seems like a quaint artifact today and it is, but you can still do many calculations without using any "mechanical" help. If you find yourself pulling out a calculator to figure out a 15 or 20 percent tip at a restaurant, you know that you are not exercising your numeric muscles. Regardless of your age, put the calculator away. If you are older and are tempted to let your adult children balance your checkbook or pay your bills, think again. A patient in her late eighties told me that continuing to handle her own financial affairs provided a regular mental challenge and even though it takes a whole morning to pay her bills and balance her accounts, she believes it is helping her stay mentally sharp. It appears to be working because she is intellectually curious and her memory for facts and events is excellent.

Many educators believe that we should keep calculators out of the classroom until students learn to do calculations without them. If we persist in allowing the use of pocket calculators or we allow students to perform math functions on their computers, numeric ability is likely to decline even further.

Verbal abilities appear to increase into one's sixties, and decline tends to start only after age sixty-five and is usually gradual. About 5 percent of people age 74–81 show enhancement of verbal ability and spatial orientation. Older people tend to notice—and note—verbal memory lapses and are often concerned when they begin to occur. The fact is, of course, that we all have lapses in verbal memory. Forgetting a name, a place, or the title of a favorite book or movie is quite common at any age. Nowadays, those still in their forties or fifties may fret about this normal forgetfulness and may even joke that the dreaded Alzheimer's is just around the corner. In fact, as discussed in the previous chapter, only a small percentage of elderly people develop senile dementia of the Alzheimer's type. In addition, verbal fluency abilities tend to decline earlier than verbal meaning skills. Thus you may not be able to recall the name of the elevator that scales the side of a mountain, while at the same time you understand when hearing about your friend's ride on one in the Alps. In other words, to forget a word is not the same as a decline in overall language skills.

One of my patients, a retired librarian, was able to classify her memory lapses based on parts of speech. For reasons we do not fully understand, lapses in verbal memory tend to involve proper and common nouns more frequently than verbs, adjectives, and adverbs. If you think about it, you are far more likely to forget the name of an acquaintance or the name of a town you once visited than the words that describe that person or place.

Broad statistical generalizations can be useful for determining situations in which declines in various abilities indicate that an abnormal degenerative process is developing. For example, a decline in verbal meaning—vocabulary—begins at about age 68 for men and 73 for women. A measurable decline of these abilities in an individual in his or her forties or fifties is not normal and should be evaluated by a physician, preferably a neurologist.

Lifestyle factors change the statistical picture. For example, if you are educated beyond high school, you can add another year to the expected age when decline begins. If you are satisfied with your life, past and present, you may be able to add on another year or two. If you are flexible, your verbal skills may not drop at all. On the other hand, a man who has low self-esteem and feels like a failure in life may begin verbal decline at age 62. His female counterpart may notice a decline in her late sixties rather than the early 70s.

Other Lifestyle Factors

A number of government agencies have combined research results and have done some comparative studies on rates of cognitive decline and dementia among a variety of populations. The purpose of the comparative studies is to look at a range of lifestyle factors and determine which, if any, can be considered risk factors. It was interesting to note that a traditional Japanese diet, which includes a significant amount of soy food products, such as miso and tofu, and green tea, was one of the few life-style factors that could be statistically linked to slight increases in rates of dementia among the elderly. The reasons for this are complex, but are related to the presence of phytoestrogens—plant estrogens—in soy products and green tea.

As you may know, there is preliminary evidence that hormone replacement therapy (HRT) given to postmenopausal women may have a protective effect against Alzheimer's disease. It is believed that the plant estrogens compete with the body's own estrogens (or estrogen introduced through hormone medications), and it is possible that phytoestrogens have a potentially adverse effect on the structure of brain cells. Paradoxically, this information comes at a time when these same plant estrogens are being discussed for their potentially protective role against breast cancer in women and prostate cancer in men, whereas HRT has been found to be ineffective in preventing cancer or heart disease.

I mention it here, but not because I intend to discourage you from using some soy products in your diet. Tofu is a high-protein meat substitute and I enjoy dishes made from tofu and other soy products. Green tea is becoming a popular drink in the United States and Europe. Much additional research is needed before definitive conclusions can be drawn about the link between specific ethnic diets and dementia. However, I would use caution in adopting a soy-protein-based diet to the exclusion of other protein sources including fish, poultry, and low-fat dairy products. Moderation is probably the best path when adding the newest "miracle" food to your diet.

The High Cost of Depression

Depression among the elderly tends to be minimized, even by family members, and if it is of some concern to you at this time,

I suggest taking the preliminary screening test for depression presented in the previous chapter. Some cases of depression may be "explained away" by pointing out that those affected have suffered many losses or have had to give up enjoyed activities. In other words, reasons for the depression may be perceived as related to circumstances, and even when it would be most helpful to do so, medical help is not sought. Much of the depression we see among the elderly responds well to anti-depressant medication because it is biological in origin. It is not character weakness or a temporary case of the "blues."

Depression often adversely affects intellectual functioning and memory. This tends to operate in a cycle in that the depressed patient loses motivation and eventually no longer tries to engage in mentally stimulating activities. Depression is not the same as grief or sadness over a loss. Most individuals move through the stages of grief and begin to live normally again. Depression interferes with normal living and may ulti-mately lead to extreme malaise and the inability to care for one's own basic needs. Individuals who experience this loss of interest and energy for day-to-day living should always be screened for depression, regardless of age.

I Can't Smell As Well As I Used To

By age 65, about 50 percent of us experience some loss in our ability to detect and identify odors. By age 80, the percentage increases to about 75 percent. Unfortunately, those who cook for the elderly in nursing homes or even in senior centers tend to be younger and they spice the food to suit their younger noses and taste buds. This loss of olfactory ability has been largely over-looked and it is unfortunate that we do not have the equivalent of hearing aids and bifocals that boost the power of the nose.

Absent head trauma or illness, the sense of smell tends to diminish gradually and the loss often goes unnoticed. However, if you find yourself enjoying food less, it may be because you no longer detect the odor and hence it is essentially tasteless. Studies have shown that older people rate stronger-smelling meats such as lamb and liver more favorably than meat with a blander odor. The elderly also tend to prefer food with softer texture, but these foods tend to be bland.

In an ideal world, the odors that the elderly population is exposed to would increase in intensity in order to make them more detectable. Food would be more heavily spiced, regardless of the texture, in order to offer a range of flavors. In your own home, be aware that as you age, your sense of smell is likely diminishing, so consciously attempt to detect fragrances around you. If your sense of smell diminishes markedly or the taste of food is altered when you are given certain medications, note this and talk with your physician about experimenting with a different medication. Begin to use odors in your home as a way of keeping a variety of smells in your life. Just as I advise you to exercise your muscles and strengthen your heart and lungs, I also believe you should exercise your nose. Practice detecting and identifying odors with the same sense of importance as when you have your vision and hearing checked. Your sense of smell is too important to ignore.

In other chapters, I have discussed the relationship of odors to learning and to mood state. That information applies to individuals of all ages. If you are faced with a task that requires your full attention, add the odor of peppermint or jasmine to your environment. If you are having trouble sleeping, try scenting your pillow with lavender or another odor that you find relaxing.

Choosing Our Role Models

Unfortunately, there are no guarantees about the aging process. We all know individuals who appeared to be in great health, yet they died prematurely or suffered greatly from a lingering illness. We may know people who appear to beat the statistical odds— the 90-year-old cigarette smoker or the 80-year-old who has a negative attitude about life, seems to enjoy being difficult, and regularly talks about death as the great escape. Yet, here they are, alive and relatively well. These individuals truly are exceptions, but not role models.

At any age, we must realize that we are charting our course for aging based on our current lifestyle. We can also aspire to living fully in the years we are here, rather than hoping to live to be 100 or even older. Look to the remarkable older people you know as role models. For me, my professor, Elizabeth Crosby, has always been a person whom I admire enormously. We all hope to be as intellectually sharp at 102 as she was.

Role models for aging can be found everywhere, sometimes in our own families and communities. In 1998, Oprah Winfrey had a special guest on her program, a man named George Dawson, who at the age of 98 decided he wanted to learn to read by the time he turned 100. The grandson of a slave, Mr. Dawson started working when he was a very young child and had never attended school. With the help of Carl Henry, a teacher in his community, Mr. Dawson achieved his goal. He was even willing to attend school with young children in order to learn the most basic literacy skills. This was undoubtedly an enriching experience for the children, who were given a chance to both help an older person reach his goal and be inspired by an elderly role model. Needless to say, it was very moving to see this gentleman reading aloud on Oprah's show. George Dawson's example shows us all that age alone should never serve as a barrier to learning and intellectual achievement.

Leave a Written Legacy

Your children and grandchildren may ask you about childhood memories or even details about family members. They may ask you to repeat old family stories or recount adventures you enjoyed as a child or young adult. Unfortunately, many families have less meaningful written information to pass on to their children. We may have many photograph albums, but we tend to write fewer letters and even financial records may be logged into a computer and discarded as soon as they are no longer needed.

Many older individuals have decided to tell their life stories, either in written form or recorded on audiotapes. This is a positive trend because it allows us to leave something tangible behind for generations to come. The idea of writing a book is not as daunting as it sounds, especially today with the technology available to inexpensively reproduce your work. In addition, the process itself is mentally stimulating and works as a memory exercise.

If you like to write, try the following:

✦ Start writing down your favorite childhood memories and stories. Put them down in random order. You can organize them in chronological order later.

✦ What world events were going on when you born? What events influenced your view of the world and made a difference in your life? What new inventions and changes have you enjoyed the most or have improved the quality of your life?

+ What were your childhood dreams?

+ What do you want your children to know about their relatives? Think about stories from their country of origin, their early jobs, and their personality quirks.

+ When your children or grandchildren ask questions about the past, jot them down and think about them later. Then, write down everything you can remember that answers the question fully.

+ What problems did you or your family face and how did you solve them?

+ What were your greatest joys in life? Do you still find great joy? Write about your most prized accomplishments and experiences.

+ Write about your most important values and life lessons. What do you want younger members of your family to remember about the era in which you lived?

After you have addressed these questions, which have no doubt triggered memories and led you to examine your relationships with other people, you can organize the material in chronological order if you wish. Some adult education centers offer classes to help you write your story. If you use a computer, it is quite easy to produce pages that can be photocopied and bound, but don't let lack of technology stop you. If necessary, write your story by hand and give it to your family members to photocopy and distribute. You will be surprised by how much information may be new, even to those closest to you.

If writing seems too daunting, then talk your story into a tape recorder. You may find yourself quite relaxed as you recount events from the past and describe people who have been important to you. You may have an adult child or grand-child who will transcribe the tapes. Then you can organize the material into a written record.

Some colleges and universities have started oral history projects in order to "capture" the wisdom of older members of the community. You can provide this service for your family— and you will likely enjoy the process yourself.

12

Nostalgia and Creating New Memories

*He was conscious of a thousand odors floating in the
air, each one connected with a thousand thoughts, and
hopes, and joys, and cares long, long forgotten."*

— Charles Dickens, *A Christmas Carol*

Nostalgia is a bittersweet yearning for the past. In psychiatry, we may call it a yearning to return home, but, more than that, it is a longing for an idealized past, or in the vernacular of the day, "a cleaned-up past." When we idealize childhood or a favorite time in our life, we edit out what is emotionally troubling or difficult to cope with, and what is left is a combination of integrated memories that we call "the past."

In a psychiatric sense, nostalgic reactions have both a positive and negative side. On the one hand, the nostalgic response may lead us to marry individuals with characteristics reminiscent of those of our parents. We may even adopt political affiliations and other attitudes because our parents held these beliefs. Unfortunately, the nostalgic urge to recreate the past explains why so many abused children marry abusive spouses. They do not do this because their childhood was happy, but rather because they try to recreate the idealized *sanitized* memories of childhood. Nostalgic responses may even contribute to the difficulty of ridding ourselves of negative attitudes and beliefs passed on to us by our parents. For example, some people retain prejudices because their parents had these beliefs, and change means rejecting a part of their childhood. Those who have had to face unpleasant childhood memories understand how difficult it can be to reject behavior and attitudes with which they grew up, while at the same time not rejecting their parents. For most of us, childhood is a mixture of memories we would just as soon forget and those we cherish. Holidays provide a good illustration of this.

Holidays, Food, Nostalgia

What are holidays if not shared efforts to recreate the past—year after year? And family arguments can become hot—not to mention completely irrational—when someone decides to change the rituals. Easter without ham? The Fourth of July barbecue without sparklers? In addition to being important to retailers, holidays usually carry both personal and cultural meaning. As a religious holiday, Easter is celebrated in numerous different ways, depending on one's ethnic background and Christian denomination. As a cultural holiday, however, the Easter bunny and egg hunts are fairly universal, yet your family may have introduced their own traditions and you might try to pass them on to your children and grandchildren.

Nowhere do personal and cultural nostalgia meet in more obvious ways than during the Thanksgiving, Christmas, and Hanukkah season. Candles and other products are specifically scented with fragrances that reflect and promote a holiday mood. Cranberry and pine scents are particularly popular around Thanksgiving and Christmas, and create a nostalgic effect in malls and other shopping areas. The odors enhance visual and auditory reminders that the holiday rituals are upon us.

In general, religious practices (and some patriotic rituals) can be viewed as an immersion in *institutionalized* nostalgia. Religious rituals may remain unchanged over millennia, thereby continually gratifying nostalgic wishes. Sometimes, when religious institutions attempt to alter or adapt beliefs or change their worship practices or rituals, they meet with great resistance. The same is true for family holiday rituals, too. When we combine family rituals with religious practices, there is an explosion, so to speak, of nostalgic desire, which explains why these special times can become such emotionally charged events for many people. Holiday stress is as much about the yearning for an idealized past as it is about demands and crammed schedules. It may be even more stressful when we attempt to suppress the painful holiday memories and replace them with happier experiences, which we then add to our storehouse of holiday memories. Yet, one of the important features of learning and memory is giving our attention to the memories we create today. Look at it this way: today's experiences create tomorrow's nostalgia.

Odors and Nostalgia

Long before scientists knew much about the sense of smell, poets and writers described its power. So many have commented on the ability of odors to evoke nostalgia that an entire volume could be filled just with their words. A straightforward description comes from Vladimir Nabokov, who said: "Nothing revives the past so completely as a smell that was once associated with it." Marcel Proust, who, perhaps more than any other writer, was intrigued by odors and nostalgia, wrote:

> When from a long distant past nothing subsists, after the people are dead, after the things are broken and scattered, still, alone, more fragile, but with more vitality, more unsubstantial, more persistent, more faithful, the smell and taste of things remain poised a long time, like souls, ready to remind us, waiting and hoping for

NOSTALGIA AND CREATING NEW MEMORIES

> *their moment, amid the ruins of all the rest; and bear*
> *unfaltering, in the tiny and almost impalpable drop of*
> *their essence, the vast structure of recollection.*

Finally, Helen Keller, a woman who could neither hear nor see, describes smell as "a potent wizard that transports us thousands of miles and across all the years we have lived."

While odors are most strongly associated with nostalgia, all the senses may be used to trigger a nostalgic response. Just look at what usually dignified 50-year-olds will do when they hear music from the 1960s. Some radio stations even specialize in "nostalgia" music, a more updated term that is replacing "golden oldies." A few children's toys remain essentially unchanged, which is why Raggedy Ann and Andy dolls and books continue to sell to each generation and Peter Rabbit stories and toys never become outdated. These products essentially satisfy the nostalgic urge and create new opportunities for nostalgic attachments in the next generation. One of the reasons that fashions seem to change in cycles, with a 1940s look popular one year and a 1970s revival emerging the next, is that the look of a long-gone decade gratifies the urge to idealize and return to the past.

Despite the importance of the other senses, the sense of smell remains the most significant in evoking the nostalgic response. And as we all know, it can be very powerful. The term we use in psychiatry is *olfactory evoked recall*, and it simply means that an odor can bring back a memory from the past. Often a vivid visual image accompanies a positive mood state. A person may detect an odor in the air and be sent off on a nostalgic reverie where a scene from the past is relived. The odor influences the limbic brain, the emotional center of the brain; the emotional response comes first and other details of the memory are "filled in" after the emotions have determined the mood. Bear in mind that the memory that is recalled is an integrated memory, not necessarily an exact recreation of the past, although it may certainly seem so real as to be exact.

Studying Nostalgia

Because we know there is a strong link between personal memories and nostalgia, our research foundation decided to take a closer look at the kinds of odors that trigger an olfactory-induced nostalgic response and olfactory-evoked recall. Are there any common odors among individuals of varying ages that evoke nostalgia?

In September 1991, we randomly selected individuals who were shopping at the Water Tower Place mall in downtown Chicago. We interviewed 989 men and women (478 men and 511 women) who were going in and out of this landmark building where many visitors to the area stop. We collected demographic data from these individuals, including the year of their birth. The majority of participants were born in the 1940s, 1950s, 1960s, and 1970s—857 in all. Three respondents were born before 1910, and the remaining 129 were born between 1910 and 1940. While most of the participants were born in the Chicago area, 45 states were represented, as well as 39 countries.

Over 85 percent of the participants displayed olfactory-evoked recall. What was most interesting were the kinds of odors that evoked recall and nostalgic responses in the different generations represented. For example, those born before the 1930s were more likely to have nostalgia induced by odors from nature—pine, hay, horses, sea air, meadows, and so forth. In those born after 1940, we saw a marked shift away from natural odors. The younger individuals—those born in the 1950s, 1960s, and 1970s —were more likely to mention Play Doh, scented markers, airplane fuel, plastic, SweetTarts, Pez, and even VapoRub.

The results are significant for a number of reasons. Consider that the younger people in our study were nostalgic for *manu-factured* odors, essentially artificial chemicals. Thirty or forty years from now, how will our environment fare if the majority of the population are nostalgic for artificial scents? How many children are being raised today without an array of natural odors around them? Probably more than we would like to admit.

We also found that the vast majority of participants reported having a happy childhood. This was a simple "yes" or "no" question, and we did not define happy childhood, nor did we ask probing questions about childhood issues. However, only one person in twelve people reported having an unhappy child-hood, and these individuals indicated that the dominant odors that induced the nostalgic response were bad odors — dog waste, sewer gas, bus fumes, and so forth. This may be negative nostalgia, but it is still induced by odor associations.

Odor Memories Provide Insight

Because odors have the power to profoundly influence our emotions and behavior, it would make sense for psychothera-pists to ask their clients about the odors that induce childhood memories. Is there a dominant odor? What is the association? I believe we can gain insight into our personality if we examine the reasons that certain odors have significant meaning for us.

Beyond that, those who develop and market products are well aware of the power of odors to stimulate a positive mood state and the nostalgic response. Both individual and collective memories are involved when products are sold partly on the basis of nostalgia. When members of a society are dissatisfied with the present, then nostalgia marketing increases because the past is idealized. When we hear people talk about the wonder-ful 1950s, the associations are with innocence and optimism.

The negative events and features of that decade seem to fade away and those who remind others that the past—any period of the past—had its downside are not appreciated for interjecting a dose of reality.

Until recently, nostalgia and the memories we have of the smells—and tastes—of the past were not given their due. However, as we learn more about the power of odors to influence behavior, we can actively create a sensory environment that promotes a positive mood state. We can use odors to influence our day-to-day learning and the quality of the memories we create.

What Memories Are You Creating Today?

Our memories influence the emotional tone of our current lives. We cherish good memories and often try to suppress our less pleasant experiences. However, little attention has been given to the actual process of creating good memories, or, put another way, creating an emotional climate that increases the opportunity for positive experiences to occur.

Our earliest memories usually involve, for better or for worse, family interactions. In addition, the memories we associate with specific people often involve odors. We remember the specific smells of our grandparent's kitchen, our older sister's cologne, or our mother's favorite powder. These odors help define the emotional quality of our relationship with these individuals. Our circle of influential individuals eventually expands. You may fondly remember a teacher's cologne, and perhaps you recall many positive experiences in her class. Others may have unpleasant associations with the cologne, and perhaps they had problems pleasing that teacher or they did poorly in the class. These individuals may still have an aversion to that cologne but not know why. The odor itself is part of the emotional tone of the memory.

In retrospect, it is difficult to study the specific childhood situations that created certain kinds of memories. The best we can do is look at common settings today, which may represent the source of either future nostalgic memories or, sadly, negative memories. The dinner table seemed like a good place to start. In a study conducted at the Smell & Taste Treatment and Research Foundation, we looked at the effects of the odor and taste of Pepperidge Farm Frozen Garlic bread on family interactions.

A Love/Hate Relationship with the Dinner Table

The fortunate among us recall pleasant interactions around the dinner table. Our parents' behavior is then linked with our memories of the food, specifically the aromas and tastes of dinner. Unfortunately, others have the opposite association. Perhaps the parents had arguments during dinner or there were many complaints about the food. Some children are constantly disciplined and the dinner table represented the place where they were belittled or even humiliated. Some children are not allowed to talk while they eat; others recall the more pleasant memory of exchanging stories about their day. Either way, the dinner table behavior can reflect the emotional atmosphere within the family and hence produce very specific memories.

Our study measured dinner table interactions of fifty families in order to see if the introduction of certain odors and tastes would alter the emotional tone. In one phase of the study, twenty-five families were provided with a spaghetti dinner that included garlic bread. The other families were provided with an identical dinner, but without the garlic bread. Our families ranged in size from two to 12 individuals, with the average family size being 3.9 persons. The 182 participants ranged from age one to age eighty-four. Ninety of our "dinner guests" were male and ninety-two were female, with the majority (72 percent) reporting that they liked the odor of garlic bread very much. Only a small percentage (about 8 percent) disliked garlic bread and the remaining group was somewhat ambivalent.

The method of recording family interactions involved using three-minute intervals during each dinner, with the first minute serving as a baseline. During the second minute, the garlic bread was presented at the table and family members could smell the aroma; during the third minute, they tasted it. Observers from our foundation recorded the number of positive and negative interactions during these three-minute intervals. The observers also noted the difference in positive or negative reactions to garlic bread.

Our 50 families had two spaghetti dinners, one with the garlic bread and one without the bread, so we had two meals for each family to use for comparison. Based on findings, we concluded that garlic bread could become a true friend of the family. The presence of garlic bread *reduced* the number of *negative* family interactions, but also *increased* the positive interactions during dinner. Individual family members were rated for their contributions to the interactions, which meant that one particularly positive or negative person would not disproportionately alter the results. In the presence of the garlic aroma and taste, the average reduction in negative interactions was 22.7 percent per minute; positive interactions increased by an average of 7.4 percent. (We specifically noted that the most reductions were in negative interactions initiated by the "dominant" male.) Older participants showed the greatest increase in pleasant interactions during the garlic bread meal. Those who liked garlic bread in the first place also showed relatively large increases in positive interactions.

More than one-third of our study participants reported an

olfactory-induced nostalgic response. The odor of garlic rarely occurs alone, but instead is linked with various kinds of food in many different ethnic dishes. The nostalgic response probably occurred because of pleasant associations of family meals. I found our results especially interesting because the odor of garlic itself is not a cosmetic odor and most people use room deodorizers to *remove* the smell of garlic from their homes. Garlic is an acceptable odor only in the right context.

Should You Create Good Memories with Garlic Bread?

We can explore many possible explanations for our garlic bread results. Perhaps most people in our fifty families liked the taste and smell of garlic bread so much that its presence led to a happier mood; most people tend to bicker less and criticize others when they're in a good mood. Our family diners, with garlic bread enhancing their mood, may have felt less confrontational or influenced by minor irritations. Some participants said the garlic bread made the meal special, which added to the pleasant mood and positive response, along with the olfactory-evoked nostalgic response. We do not know if the aroma of garlic exerts a direct effect on the brain and therefore influences behavior by changing brain wave activity or brain chemistry.

This study shows the potential importance of aromas and food when we create experiences that lead to elevated mood and positive interactions, which in turn have at least a subtle effect on creating associations and memories. Would other foods produce similar results? Since the smell and taste of garlic is pleasant only in the context of food and meals, it cannot be studied without interference from other variables. On the other hand, we have studied green apple, cucumber, pumpkin pie, and other food odors, which are considered pleasant, even without the presence of the food itself.

Studying Family Interactions

Family life is one of the most important influences in childhood. Despite the exposure to school, social activities, and television, we learn much about human interaction within our families. Family meals often set the tone for the quality of interaction among family members. It is unfortunate, but true, that many people do not have pleasant childhood memories of family meals eaten in a warm atmosphere. Even when family life is working fairly well, meals are often rushed occasions with over-stressed parents presiding. These are not the conditions under which positive memories are created.

The purpose behind the purpose, so to speak, of our study involves the process of creating pleasant memories. We often forget that memories are cumulative and every day we create new memories. What we do today and how we behave today constitute the memories we will have tomorrow. Our research with garlic bread is important only if we take seriously the idea that the atmosphere, including the odors of the foods we serve, can influence our interactions. I hope that our study stimulates more research into this area of family life.

I also hope that it reminds you that the atmosphere in your home today is creating the memories that your children carry with them for life. This is not meant to be a "guilt trip," but simply my way of emphasizing the importance of being conscious of how we interact with those we love. Too often, we forget how important even a simple odor can be in elevating mood and improving communication.

How Will You Remember Today?

The information in this chapter is meant to heighten your consciousness about the relationship between today's activities and behavior and the memories you and your family will share years from now. I leave you with two suggestions that not only will help you enhance the quality of your life today, but also will provide a tangible way to trigger memories in the future. The first also has practical value in improving your memory.

Keep a family journal

Most people associate journaling with introspection or private writing, but a family journal may be little more than recording your family's activities and impressions of your current family life. In a sense, you are writing a family history *as you live it*. Later, if you decide to write your life story for your family, these journals will avoid all the speculation about what year particular events occurred.

I don't discourage you from keeping a personal journal if you wish, but I suggest creating a family journal, too. In this age of e-mail communication and computers, most of us have few handwritten letters or journals to refer to when we want to reflect on the past. We may even become frustrated when we try to remember details about our first apartment or the color of the kitchen in the first home we purchased. Many of us keep photo albums, but we lose the immediate record of our impressions of the events. Pictures tell one part of a story, but your written record completes the memory of the experience. As your children learn to read and write, they may want to add to the journal, too.

Create a family memory ritual that leaves something tangible behind

You may have special rituals around holidays and other events, but I suggest maintaining a sense of permanency about the ritual. The best way to describe what I mean is to tell you about a ritual we have in our family. Starting with the birth of our first child, I decided that on each Father's Day I would write my children a letter and tell them the things about them that stand out in my mind. I want to give them a sense of the atmosphere around them as each year passes. The easiest way to describe this is to show you the letter I wrote on Father's Day 2001.

> *To my children on Father's Day, June 17, 2001,*
> *I love you all.*
> *To Noah* [our one-year-old], *I love the way you smile at me, the way you wave bye-bye, and the light in your eyes when you hear your toy fish singing.*
> *To Camryn* [our two-year-old], *I love the way you scream when we play monster and hide-and-go-seek, your cute eyes at "half-mast" when you suck your thumb as you're about to fall asleep, your exuberance when you chase your older brother and sister and try to keep up with their play, and your future career choice, to be Cinderella.*
> *To Jack* [our four-year-old], *I love your puppy-dog enthusiasm, your care and concern for your younger brother and sister, and your playful nature.*
> *To Marissa* [our eight-year-old], *I love your kind and gentle heart, the way you try to fool me when you disobey (like drinking soda when I said "water only"), I love your care and concern for everyone's feelings.*
> *I feel so blessed to have the best children in the world. Thank you for a wonderful Father's Day.*
> *Love, Daddy*

This type of letter represents just one idea, and you're welcome to use it if you believe it will help preserve precious memories, your own and your children's. The small events in our children's lives tend to fade with time, and most of us tend to forget the little things our children do that bring us joy. I also write this letter because I believe it will help my children gain access to their childhood memories.

Beyond the Facts of Memory

Most information presented about memory and learning speculates about and emphasizes the practical issues, and that is true for this book, too. Understanding basic brain functions, improving our memory for names, enhancing our ability to concentrate, recognizing the consequences of malodors on learning, and striving to maintain and expand intellectual abilities over a lifetime are worthy pursuits.

In the end, however, the emotional tones of your memories are critical in determining if you live happily or unhappily every day. As a psychiatrist, I am sure that the memories of the people you have known in your life are far more important for your quality of life than the quantity of information you have accumulated over the years. When you consider improving your ability to learn and remember, try first to improve the emotional tone of the memories you are creating every day.

Bibliography

Hirsch, A.R., Johnston, L.H. Odors and learning. *Journal of Neurology, Orthopedic Medicine and Surgery,* 1996; 17:119-126.

Hirsch, A.R., Colavincenzo, M.L. Olfactory assessment of neurologic inpatients. [paper]

Hirsch, A.R., Gruss, J.J. Human male sexual response to olfactory stimuli. *Journal of Neurology, Orthopedic Medicine and Surgery,* 1999; 19:14-19.

Hirsch, A.R. Scent and sexual arousal. Could fragrance help relieve sexual dysfunction? *Medical Aspects of Human Sexuality,* 1998; 1:3:9-12

Hirsch, A.R., Colavincenzo, M.L. The Alcohol Sniff Test compared with the University of Pennsylvania Smell Identification Test. *Chemical Senses,* 2000; 25:5.

Hirsch, A.R., Gruss, J.J. Ambient odors in the treatment of claustrophobia: A pilot study. *Journal of Neurology, Orthopedic Medicine and Surgery,* 1998; 18:98-103.

Hirsch, A.R., Colavincenzo, M.L. The effects of odors on Physiological Measurements of Anxiety. [abstract] 46th Annual Meeting, Academy of Psychosomatic Medicine, 1999.

Hirsch, A.R. Sensory Marketing. *The International Journal of Aromatherapy,* 1993; 5:1:21-23.

Hirsch, A.R. Effects of ambient odors on slot-machine usage in a Las Vegas casino. *Psychology & Marketing,* 1995; 12:7:585-594.

Hirsch, A.R. Negative health effects of malodors in the environment: A brief review. *Journal of Neurology, Orthopedic Medicine and Surgery,* 1998; 18:43-45.

DeCook, C.A., Hirsch, A.R. Anosmia due to inhalational zinc: A case report. *Chemical Senses,* 2000; 25:5.

Hirsch, A.R., Bissell, G. Effects of acute alcohol inebriation on human olfaction: A preliminary report. *Journal of Neurology, Orthopedic Medicine and Surgery,* 1998; 18:114-121.

Hirsch, A.R., Zavala G. Long term effects on the olfactory system of exposure to hydrogen sulphide. *Occupational and Environmental Medicine,* 1999; 56:284-287.

Hirsch, A.R., Kang, C. The effect of inhaling green apple fragrance to reduce the severity of migraine: A pilot study. *Headache Quarterly,* 1998; 9:159-163.

Hirsch, A.R. Nostalgia: A neuropsychiatric understanding. *Advances in Consumer Research,* 1992; 19:390-395.

Hirsch, A.R. Effects of garlic bread on family interactions. *Psychosomatic Medicine,* 2000; 62:1:103-104.

Products & Services
Dr. Alan Hirsch

Smell or Taste Problem

If you or any members of your family have difficulties with reduced, odd, or increased ability to smell or taste and you have questions, I would be happy to speak with you. You can contact me at:

Alan R. Hirsch, M.D.
Smell & Taste Treatment and Research Foundation
845 North Michigan Avenue, Suite 990w
Chicago, Illinois 60611
312-938-1047
dr.hirsch@core.com

To find out more about the Smell & Taste Treatment and Research Foundation, log onto www.smellandtaste.org.

Toys to Enhance Learning

A line of fifteen different toys, odorized to intensify a child's learning, has been developed by Baby Boom. Called "Smart Scents," these toys are currently available in many retail chains and toy stores. To locate the store nearest you, log onto www.beteshgroup.com.

Weight Loss

The book, *Scentsational Weight Loss,* Fireside Books, NY, 1997, is available at bookstores, and online at www.amazon.com or www.barnesandnoble.com. It is also available through our website, www.smellandtaste.org and by calling (312) 938-1047. (ISBN 0-684-84566-0)

The Secret to Using Aroma for Sexual Arousal

The book, *Scentsational Sex,* Element Books, Inc., MA, 1998, is available at bookstores, and online at www.amazon.com or www.barnesandnoble.com. It is also available through our website, www.smellandtaste.org and by calling (312) 938-1047. (ISBN 1-86204-241-1)

Discover Your True Personality

The book, *What Flavor Is Your Personality? Discover Who You Are By Looking at What You Eat,* Sourcebooks, Inc., IL, 2001, is available at bookstores, and online at www.amazon.com or www.barnesandnoble.com. It is also available through our website, www.smellandtaste.org and by calling (312) 938-1047. (ISBN 1-57071-647-1)